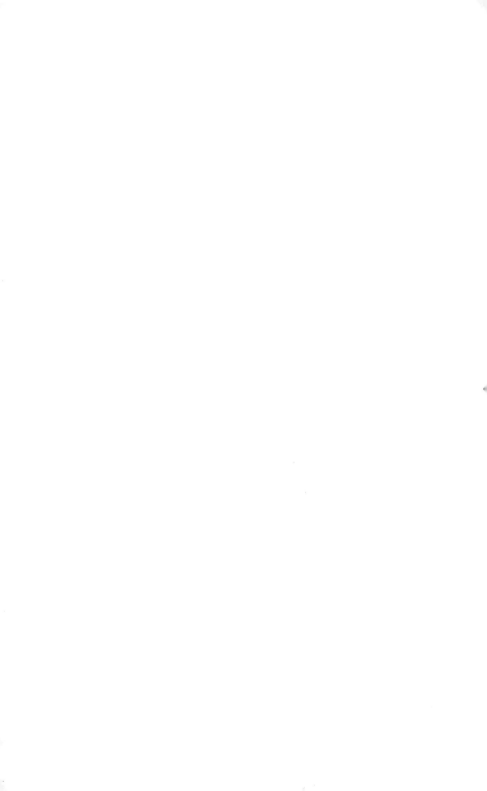

DIE YOUNG WITH ME

A Memoir

ROB RUFUS

TOUCHSTONE

New York London Toronto Sydney New Delhi

Touchstone
An Imprint of Simon & Schuster, Inc.
1230 Avenue of the Americas
New York, NY 10020

First Touchstone hardcover edition September 2016

TOUCHSTONE and colophon are registered trademarks of
Simon & Schuster, Inc.

For information about special discounts for bulk purchases,
please contact Simon & Schuster Special Sales at 1-866-506-1949
or business@simonandschuster.com.

The Simon & Schuster Speakers Bureau can bring authors to
your live event. For more information or to book an event,
contact the Simon & Schuster Speakers Bureau at 866-248-3049
or visit our website at www.simonspeakers.com.

Interior design by Kyle Kabel

Manufactured in the United States of America

10 9 8 7 6 5 4 3 2 1

Library of Congress Cataloging-in-Publication Data

Names: Rufus, Rob, author.
Title: Die young with me : a memoir / by Rob Rufus.
Description: New York : Touchstone Books, 2016.
Identifiers: LCCN 2016005363| ISBN 9781501142611 (hardcover) |
ISBN 9781501142628 (pbk.)
Subjects: LCSH: Rufus, Rob. | Punk rock musicians—United States
—Biography. | Cancer—Patients—Biography.
Classification: LCC ML420.R8932 A3 2016 | DDC 782.42166092
—dc23 LC record available at http://lccn.loc.gov/2016005363

ISBN 978-1-5011-4261-1
ISBN 978-1-5011-4263-5 (ebook)

Certain names and identifying characteristics have been changed,
including those of the doctors I saw in West Virginia.

For my brother

CONTENTS

CONTENTS

We'll take on the midnight hour
In those bitchin' black leather soles,
We'll go where time won't reach us
I comb my hair back before I go,
Feel that dull blade in your hand
My sworn blood brother, my only friend,
We'll meet again
Somewhere
But man, I don't know when . . .

There are no soft farewells or sweet partings
There are no rested bones
Just stacks of empty cards from empty friends
That never show,
Stained white rooms radiate the long black shadow of wasted days
As my soft sunken eyes grow dim
Inside some stranger's face . . .

But once, I dreamed I was running through hospital halls
I was blowing off the doors,
You can pull these needles from my arms
Man, I don't hurt no more,
I dreamed I was running through hospital halls
I was blowing off the doors . . .

And then I woke up alone
Beneath fluorescent lights,
Like a love unknown
Like a ghost in the night

Don't you want to die young?

DIE YOUNG WITH ME

SIDE A

Revolution rock, it is a brand-new rock,
A bad, bad rock, this here revolution rock . . .

—The Clash
("Revolution Rock")

ONE

Unknown Road

1

I heard it before I saw it.

We were standing beneath the marquee of the movie theater, trying to decide where to skate, when I noticed the muffled sound of music—hard rock music—coming from somewhere on the street. Nat heard it too. It was in the air all around us, floating in the heavy purple sky among the smell of rotting fish.

Paul saw the sign—DAVIDSON'S MUSIC—above one of the usually vacant storefronts that lined Fourth Avenue. We'd never had a real record store in Huntington. No one seemed to have much throwaway money in our small little river town, so cassettes and CDs seemed frivolous, and weren't exactly in high demand. The only time I bought music was at Sears with my parents; or if I ordered by mail from magazine tear-outs. We grabbed our boards and went over to check it out.

There were no customers inside. There were no employees either, as far as I could tell. But there was music. Man, there was music! It came blaring from some hidden stereo. Shelves of vinyl records wrapped the store like a moat—in the middle was an island of CDs, *hundreds* of them. The walls were covered in posters of rock bands, black-light skulls, pot leaves, bikini wet dreams.

It was rock 'n' roll in freaky 3-D vision.

The music was too loud for me to speak. The entire store seemed electric, as if the walls themselves were vibrating. I felt, for an instant, like I was vibrating too—like I'd stepped into some sort of conduit, the insides buzzing with raw fucking power.

I'd never been anywhere like this before.

West Virginia summers are brutal. The heat rises up from the south, and by July the Ohio River seems like it's about to boil over, engulfing our town in the faint smell of catfish. Big fucking whiskered catfish.

In fact, the only thing that smelled worse than the river that summer was us.

We skateboarded downtown every day. The heavy air blew against us as we roared down cement streets like something out of a suburban nightmare. We weaved through cars like psycho-banshees, horrifying drivers, hobos, and adults on their lunch break.

At least that's what I liked to think. In truth, I doubt our little gang looked like much more than we were—a handful of bored thirteen-year-olds looking for a way to kill time.

The lanky one with the acne was Tyson. He was the smart one, not that it mattered. Peter had the bowl cut, and was the one kid in our group fatter than me. The mean-looking one, the one with the three-inch scar on his forehead, was Paul. Paul lived three streets down from me in a two-room apartment he shared with his disabled mom, adult brother, and nine cats.

Then, of course, there was my twin brother—Nat, my opposite number, my eternal partner in crime. Nat and I weren't just physically identical—short, chubby, blue-eyed Hitler Youth rejects—we had the exact same interests and opinions about literally everything. In fact, most people didn't even bother learning our names. They referred to us as one entity—"the twins."

I never minded too much.

Our crew had banded together sometime during our seventh-grade year—we didn't have much in common, besides being perpetually uninvited to life. We were on the outside of something, and we knew it. That's how we found each other. It was as if we'd been wilting on the same damn wall.

So that summer, we took up skateboarding. We took up slacking. We took up *rebelling*—our small-town version of it, anyway. We started doing all the things that outcasts are supposed to do.

We claimed ownership of the streets and sidewalks of Huntington. We bombed hills, we ollied stairs, we ruined benches and ledges all over town—we skated our way through the heat, as puberty rang from our bodies like a sponge on the sidewalk.

It was exhausting, the heat. It made it hard to enjoy yourself. It was tough to fight the urge to go back home, crank the AC, and watch shitty daytime TV until our parents got home.

By the end of June we were really struggling. We forced ourselves out into the streets. The reign of our skater gang wouldn't have lasted much longer if it weren't for that record store opening up.

Davidson's Music—a home away from home. A stopping point. A destination. A sanctuary from the fiery hell of a sweat-stained Appalachian summer.

Going to the record store became part of our summer routine. We rarely had money to spend on music, but anytime we needed a break from the heat we would haunt the aisles of Davidson's, flipping through the shrink-wrapped jewel cases with idle intent.

Eventually, employees manifested. There was Chris, a white guy with dreadlocks who was always reading magazines behind the register. The other guy, Egor, was six feet tall, with stringy black hair running down to where his ass should have been. Egor's face was covered in metal—rings and pins stuck out of his nose, eyebrows, ears, lips, chin, and who knows where else. I don't know if he actually *worked* there, but Egor was always around.

We never met anyone by the name of Davidson. It was always just these two guys. I don't know where they came from, or why. They looked like musicians, but weren't. They looked like skaters too, but they didn't skate. Back then, they woulda been called "slackers"—except I couldn't square that, because I only saw them at work.

To me, they just kinda looked like two guys who didn't give a fuck.

And *that* made a big impression on me. These almost-slackers seemed like the coolest dudes who'd ever lived in our town. I wanted to read the magazines they were reading, use the slang they were using, wear the clothes they were wearing. I wanted to find out what metal shit they stuck in their face and stick it in *my* face—these two weirdos were the gatekeepers to something special.

I knew it, even if they never did.

Anytime I had money to spend, I would ask what they were listening to. Chris usually guided me to the cassettes (they were cheaper) and ran through the new releases. He said it was a great year for rock; he called it the summer of loud. Helmet, Metallica, Smashing Pumpkins, Weezer, Bush, Nirvana, Rage Against the Machine—anything he recommended, I bought. By the time my parents told me that we were going to a family reunion in Richmond, Virginia, over Fourth of July weekend, Nat and I were in the first stages of having a pretty killer music collection.

We packed all of our tapes for the drive. Dad drove slowly, blasting Van Morrison, Jackson Browne, and then Van Morrison again. Nat and I sat in the backseat with the stack of cassettes between us. The headphones of our Walkmen never left our ears.

* * *

The reunion was held at our uncle Tony's house, right outside the Richmond city limits. It was a pretty good time, all in all, and seeing my relatives meant scoring some late-birthday cash.

I spent most of that first day with Mammaw Rufus, who loved to freak us out with overly graphic stories of the insane asylum where she worked as a ward nurse. But by the time evening rolled around, I was feeling pretty damn bored.

The adults sat at the kitchen table drinking Johnnie Walker and playing Rook. Pretty normal Richmond behavior. By ten o'clock the place seemed more like a saloon—shit-talking bourbon yells filled the kitchen. Uncle Carl's cigarette ash piled on the linoleum floor. Nat and I were just standing around.

We were supposed to sleep in our cousin Anthony's room, which was directly downstairs, in the basement. I couldn't remember the last time I'd seen Anthony— maybe Christmas, four or five years earlier. I was nervous of what he'd think of me. He was only a few years older than us, but when you're a teenager, a few years is a lifetime.

Except we'd been at the house all day, and I hadn't seen my cousin once.

Mammaw's team won the hand—again. Aunt Rose went out for cigarettes, Uncle Tony shuffled the deck, and Dad refilled the drinks.

"Fuck this," Nat mumbled.

He went down the stairs to the basement. A few seconds later, he was back.

"Dude, you *have* to see this place."

I almost fell as he dragged me down the stairs.

The basement looked less like a bedroom and more like a separate apartment. It stretched the width of the entire house, with its own door leading to the carport—offering Anthony a level of freedom that I never knew kids could possess.

Photographs were taped to the walls: class photos, a few pictures of snowboarders, some dark pictures from parties or concerts—I recognized Anthony at once. He had that same Rufus smile and jaw.

More important than the photos of my cousin were all the photos of girls—not foldout centerfolds or *Sports Illustrated* shit, I mean *real* girls.

My cousin in a tux, a too-thin blonde with her hands on a pillar beside him. *Here*—Anthony's arm around a bikini brunette. *More*—snapshots of all kinds of girls, wallet-size proof of *something*. I wondered if he was dating any of them. I wondered if he dated *all* of them. Maybe he traded the pictures like baseball cards.

"Bones Brigade," Nat said, behind me.

He was looking at an old-school Powell skateboard deck, nailed above Anthony's bed. I broke off from the girls and checked out the rest of the room.

There were a few other skateboards—most looked broken—parked against walls or leaning on furniture. Two unmatched bookshelves lined the far wall. They were spray-painted black, and covered in dozens of stickers.

There were no books on the shelves—only music.

The bottom shelves were reserved for vinyl; dog-eared rows of albums ran straight across. On the middle two shelves, CDs were stacked carelessly, many not even in cases. The top shelves held better-organized stacks of tapes, 7" vinyl, and five cases of unopened blank cassettes.

He had more music than anyone I'd ever met. I wanted to start digging through it but was afraid if I tried, the entire stack would crumble.

I plopped down on the threadbare couch. It faced a big TV with large stereo speakers on each side of it. Nat crouched down below it, where the stereo console was. It had a turntable, *four* cassette players, and a *six*-CD changer.

"Who the fuck is our cousin, again?" Nat said.

He sat down beside me and faced the blank screen.

I woke to the sound of a door slamming shut. I'd dozed off at some point in the night. I had no clue what time it was. The drunken jeers from upstairs were replaced with silence.

I rubbed my eyes and looked toward the carport door.

"What up, cuz," Anthony said. He tossed his keys onto the coffee table in front of me.

My cousin looked different than I remembered. He'd grown into his features, and had an apathetic handsomeness that made me instantly jealous. He unzipped his black leather jacket. Buttons and safety pins ran down the collar. On him, a leather jacket in July made perfect sense.

We gave each other an awkward hug. Anthony smelled like stale beer. He sat down on the coffee table, facing us. We made small talk about the reunion.

I asked him about the girls on the wall. Anthony got lost in each one, going into serious specifics—who did which drugs, who had the best body, which girl was willing to do what (and if so, how she did it). It was goddamn impressive.

Anthony got up and turned on his stereo. The music sounded so distorted that I wondered if a speaker was busted.

"Man," he said, "there were some serious babes at our show *tonight*, though. I mean, damn . . . some wild-looking chicks."

"What kind of show?" Nat asked. "A concert?"

"Yeah, my band played downtown at Alley Kats. I figured my dad told y'all."

"You're a musician?" I said.

Anthony laughed. "I didn't say *that*. Shit, musicians play clarinet. I said I was in a band."

"Oh," I said, clearly confused.

"Yeah, I play bass in a band called Witness. We are kind of like Inquisition mixed with Avail, and a few songs sound more like 7 Seconds. You know, kinda Youth of Today–ish."

I nodded. Nat nodded. Neither of us had any idea what the fuck he was talking about.

"You guys dig those bands?" he asked us.

I was about to lie, but Nat told him no.

"What about Ann Beretta? Or Crass. Or like, Social D, or the Misfits?" Their names were as unfamiliar and dumb-sounding as the first bands he mentioned.

Again, Nat told him no.

"Shit man," he said, "don't you guys listen to punk at all?"

"I dunno." I shrugged.

Anthony sighed. He stumbled off the table and began rummaging through his records, tossing them out of order onto the floor. Nat and I sat perfectly still.

Anthony held up a record. The cover was a black-and-white photo of four dudes in leather jackets standing against a brick wall. The band name above them was written in neon pink.

"What about the Ramones?" he asked. "There's no way you've never even listened to the Ramones."

Nat took the album. He inspected it like it was some new technology he wasn't sure how to use.

"I've heard of them," he said, "I think."

"Fuck! I thought y'all skated! How can you skate and *not* listen to punk?"

We didn't know.

Anthony shook his head and sat back down on the table. He sighed again.

"Well, goddamn, I guess that's what happens when you live in West Virginia, huh?"

We guessed it was.

The three of us sat silent. The world outside was quiet and sleeping.

"Well," I said, nervously, "why don't you *fucking* play us some."

"Ha!" Anthony laughed. "There's that Rufus blood. Fuck yeah!"

He jumped up off the table and went back to the bookshelves. He pulled a cassette tape out of a pile.

"This band's the shit," he said. "It's *killer* jams for skating."

"What is it?" I asked.

"*Unknown Road*—by Pennywise."

He pressed play. He cranked the stereo volume, oblivious to the adults who were sleeping upstairs.

The guitar came in first. It sounded like a chain saw cutting through my ears. Then, all of a sudden, the entire song blasted into the room at full force. I'd never heard drums played so *fast*—they sounded like someone hitting trash cans with a baseball bat. The song had so much speed that I might have thought it was a joke if my heart wasn't pounding.

The singer sort of yelled, sort of talked over the music.

I couldn't tell what the words were, but I could tell that he believed them. He sounded too pissed off to care about something as dumb as singing. He just wanted to be heard.

It is hard for me to describe, even now. I'd never heard *anything* like punk rock before—it was like all the bands I normally listened to, except on overdrive. It was raw. And it was bad, but in the very best way.

"This is awesome!" Nat yelled over the chorus. "This band is fucking *awesome!*"

I rocked back and forth, not sure what to do. I needed to move. I wanted to skate, Anthony was right—I wanted to go fast.

As the songs sped up, I got more excited. I felt like throwing the coffee table through the fucking TV. I wanted to go *fast*. I wanted to go down the unknown road.

I couldn't make out the words, but I felt like I knew what he was yelling about.

We sat in the basement all night. Anthony flipped from cassette to vinyl, CD to CD, then back to tape. He was the DJ of our future, and he was too drunk to know.

I never got off the couch. I bounced on the dead springs like I had the shakes. Nat sat beside me, looking through liner notes. The stereo played on.

The Ramones, the Descendents, the Humpers, Bad Religion, the Misfits, Minor Threat, Strife, Face to Face, TSOL, Screeching Weasel, Rancid, the Clash—all of the songs were high-speed. Every singer sounded angry; even the love songs had an undertone of rage.

Nat and I passed the liner notes back and forth. The

bands in the photos looked different from any I'd seen on TV. The Misfits looked like Satan worshippers. The Descendents looked like four-eyed dorks. The guitarist in Poison Idea looked too fat to stand up onstage. *God, I* thought, *some of these bands are even more tragic than me.*

Which, of course, made them the coolest bands in the world.

These were musicians I could relate to—I didn't feel so different from any of these guys. I felt in time with their beat. It connected with me so instantly that it seemed instinctual.

The guitars played the same chords over and over. The drummers pounded—*babababababababap!*—like madmen. The singers screamed or sneered or whined or mumbled—it all connected with me.

I felt the power in it.

Music like this had the power to change people. It had the power to scare people. I knew that from the start. But it didn't scare my brother. And it didn't scare me.

From that first chord, to my last chord, it never scared me.

Up until that night, I'd felt like I was on the outside of my own life. Forever out of step at school, in the neighborhood, even with my own family. But hearing that music, seeing those photos, reading the lyrics—they made it seem okay to be out of place. These bands made it seem *cool.*

This was it. Even if I didn't say so, I knew. Now I had something to relate to. I had something to claim, and I had something that was willing to claim me. I finally had a flag to fly under—one perfect and fucked up and black.

* * *

We listened to music until four in the morning. Anthony spent those last hours sitting on his knees, surrounded by cellophane and blank tapes. Whenever we *really* liked a record, he dubbed over a bootleg copy for us.

We didn't wake up until way past noon.

Anthony drove us into Carytown, a neighborhood on the north end of Richmond, where there were skate shops, bars, tattoo parlors, and record stores. My cousin was hip to it all.

The freaks, the druggies, and the punks were all there in the flesh. We passed a gang of Mohawked kids with neon hair and black T-shirts. I saw a group of tattooed guys sitting on the stoop of a town house smoking cigarettes. Everyone we passed on the street could have walked straight outta Anthony's record collection.

More weirdos loitered outside of Plan 9 Music. I was careful not to bump any of them as I followed Anthony inside.

Plan 9 was the size of a warehouse. Large windows ran three stories high, giving everything inside a natural glow. There were *thousands* of records, CDs, tapes, mags, and comic books within my reach. In the back were cases of patches, posters, T-shirts, and buttons. Shit, this place made Davidson's Music seem like a joke.

I was a silent observer.

Who wore what? Who bought what? Who talked how, and why? I spied on the entire store, picking up what I could.

We pooled our birthday money together, ready to blow

it all on stacks of cassettes, black T-shirts, and issues of *Alternative Press* and *Maximum Rocknroll*.

We stood at the register behind a long line of record shoppers.

Nat flipped through the magazines, studying them like they were punk rock syllabi. I just studied the checkout girl.

She had tattoos—leopard spots running halfway down her left arm. Her hair and her lips were a matching bright pink. Two silver rings stuck out from her bottom lip, weighing it down in a permanent pout.

The line inched forward. I focused on her lips. When the light reflected off the rings, they looked almost like fangs.

She rang me up and took my money. I couldn't look away from the vampire lip.

"Solid choices, man," she said, smiling and handing me my bag.

"*Fuck yeah,* man," I squeaked back.

I tripped over myself on the way out the door.

*　　*　　*

The next morning, we left for home. I dreaded going back. Our friends, our record store, the town itself—everything seemed even smaller now.

I'd had my first taste of counterculture, and it lingered in my mouth. Huntington didn't even have any culture *to* counter! I wanted to stay in Richmond. I wanted to be part of *this*!

But as soon as we pulled out of my uncle's driveway,

the city faded quickly away. I sat in the backseat of the car, watching blurry colors of brick and black blend into a sea of endless green. Trees ebbed and flowed on the mountains around us. The interstate cut through them like a huge cement snake.

Soon, we were back in nowhere.

I looked over at my brother beside me. His headphones were on. His eyes were shut, but he was awake. He was nodding, just barely, with the music. He tapped the empty *Brain Drain* jewel case on his knee.

He didn't look depressed. He didn't mind that we were going home. He didn't care where we were going. He was already gone.

TWO

My Basement Life

1

Nat wanted to transform our basement into a carbon copy of the one in Richmond. I considered it a useless cause—mainly because our basement was complete shit.

Stained carpet was glued unevenly to the corners of the floor. It stopped suddenly, as if the contractor had simply run out of material. There was an old love seat in one corner. A dusty shelf hung above it, and a single-pane window above that. Like I said—shit.

But Nat was convinced that the basement was a key factor in the power of the music. He said it sounded better when it was a private thing.

So that first week home from Richmond, he stayed in the basement for hours, killing the last days of summer vacation. He angled the love seat into the corner. He put his small boom box beside it, and taped up pages of liner notes around it. He plastered the rest of the walls with the torn pages of skateboard and music magazines.

I was really impressed by his progress, until all the tapes, CDs, and magazines began disappearing from my bedroom.

I went down to ask him about it. He was sitting on the floor in front of the stereo and poring over one of Dad's yellow legal pads.

"What are you writing?" I asked.

"See all these liner notes? I was going through them, ya know, and got to reading the 'thank you' sections—they all have one. The bands always thank other bands, so I've been writing down all the band names that I don't recognize. I figure once we get some funds, we can go to Davidson's and see if they carry any of them."

"Dude," I said, "that is fucking genius."

He handed me the list. There were probably sixty bands on it. I'd never seen him put so much work into *anything*.

"Hey," I said, "speaking of—where are the tapes you took outta my room? I wanted to listen to *Everything Sucks*."

Nat nodded to the shelf beneath the window. "I figured we can keep them all down here from now on. They're in ABC order, though—don't fuck them up."

I had to stand on the love seat to reach the shelf. I couldn't see many—just Nirvana, Everclear, and the treasures we'd brought back from Richmond. There were only about ten CDs total, in a neat little row with cassettes stacked three deep beside them.

"Where are the rest of our records?" I asked.

"That stuff from before, it didn't belong down here, man. It's out in the alley."

* * *

Bon Jovi. Boyz II Men. Weird Al. Ace of Base. The *Lion King* soundtrack. There were dozens of CDs and tapes, broken and blackened, melded together in the alley behind our garage. Nat had burnt them all.

Cusswords and anarchy signs had been carved on the backs of CDs. Spools of tape lay dead in the alley like discarded snakeskins. He'd arranged the pile neatly atop his old Boy Scout kerchief. Baseball cards and a Troll doll seemed to have been used as accelerants. A tin of lighter fluid was propped against the garage.

It was all represented in the pile, everything we'd once claimed. The sports we'd tried—and failed—to play. The groups we'd tried to join. The music we'd bought mindlessly, without even knowing if we actually liked it. Different styles and phases we'd tried on for size—all there in the pile.

What would Anthony have said about Nat's old Aerosmith tape? What would vampire girl think of my Hootie & the Blowfish CD? It didn't matter anymore. The slate had to be cleared. Burning meant that.

Now, for once, we were committed.

Nat walked up behind me. We stood there looking down at the rubble.

"The crazy thing is, it only took one match."

2

It was too hot out to skate, so Paul and the guys started hanging out in our basement with us. We played them our punk records, introducing them to the music the way our cousin had. They reacted almost as strongly as me.

Some days, if any of us had cash, we made the death-march up to the record store to try and mark another band off Nat's list. Since we were their only steady customers,

Chris and Egor began ordering more punk music from their record distributors—but if they did manage to get a punk album in, it was only one copy. Meaning whichever one of us bought it did so with the knowledge that he'd have to dub copies for everyone else.

Mom was worried that we spent too much time in the basement. It was unhealthy, she said, to listen to that noise all day instead of being in the fresh air. That's what she called it—*noise*.

But it was all we wanted to do. I wanted to have the same attitude that these punk rock bands had. I wanted to have the balls to take on the world the way they did.

So, as the sun shined through that small window, we sat down there, my brother and my friends and I, playing the same records over and over and over again, like members of a cult who were trying to brainwash themselves.

3

School was harder on all of us now.

Paul got beat up the third week of school because he "dressed like a fucking faggot"—it was four guys, behind the bleachers after football practice. Paul didn't dress any different than he had the year before, except for a chain he now wore as a bracelet (like the guitarist in Rancid did). None of the fucks responsible got in trouble.

It wasn't like we'd suddenly become mutants. We wore a few chains and buttons, maybe some band T-shirts, but that's all. Otherwise, we were the same boring-ass white boys we'd always been.

But the other kids treated us differently. It was as if they sensed we no longer had an urge to fit their definition of "cool," so we got treated with a special kind of disdain.

Whenever the final school bell rang, my muscles instantly loosened. I'd rush to my locker, maneuvering through the halls as if I was scared I might get trapped inside the building. After what had happened to Paul, I started using the side exit.

The guys still came by our house most days, to hang out in the basement with Nat and me. We sat around until dusk, talking shit and replaying whatever album we were hooked on at the time.

But whenever my parents got home, the guys split.

Our dinner table was silent now. Mom didn't know what to say to us anymore, and we didn't know what to say to her. School had made me more sensitive than I used to be. Any question or comment that came from my parents felt only like a judgment, a continuation of the vibes I got from my classmates and teachers.

Once the table was cleared and the shitty sitcoms came on, we could all relax. Mom and Dad watched the TV, and I went up to my bedroom. I always locked the door.

I put on my headphones and strapped my Walkman to my pants. Then I stood in front of the mirror. When the tape came on, I would shred the air guitar, and sing to my reflection with the showmanship and passion of a goddamn pro. I did it for hours some nights, rocking through albums like I was filming my own music video. I got so immersed in it that by the time I quit I'd be sweating.

I don't know why I never thought of playing music for real. I was staring at the possibility every night—right there in front of me. And by the time my private concerts were over, the bullshit of my day was all lost in the feedback.

* * *

One day after school, Nat told me that we were starting a band.

"Who is?" I asked.

He shrugged. "Me. You. Whoever. Who *cares*? Us, dude!"

"We don't play instruments."

"Sean does."

"Who?"

"*Sean*, man, shit," Nat said, annoyed. "He just transferred here this week. His dad works for the railroad or something. He's in my English class. He fucking plays guitar, dude!"

"Is he any good?"

"Jesus, man, it's *punk*—who cares if he's good?"

"Well," I said, "what am I going to play?"

"Drums."

"*Drums?* I don't know."

"I do," Nat said. "Because we are the only ones who even *have* a basement. The other guys can't fit a drum kit into those shoe boxes they live in. Besides, I'm playing bass. So we need a drummer."

"Why do you get to play bass?"

"*Because* it was my idea—and because I called it first."

I sighed. "Well, who would sing?"

"Maybe Tyson, Paul, or Peter. I don't know yet. Whoever is ballsy enough to get onstage and do it, I guess. It doesn't matter who sings."

"Well, how are we gonna get instruments, or shows, or . . ."

"Do you not wanna do it?"

"I mean *of course* I want to do it."

"Well, then shut the fuck up," he said.

I shut the fuck up.

* * *

Nat promised he'd talk to our parents about it. If they could spring the money for some instruments, we would do odd jobs until they were paid back. I didn't think they'd ever go for it, especially Dad. A college wrestling champion turned Vietnam vet, our father had been given the awkward job of raising two sloth-like apples who couldn't have fallen farther from his tree. Our off-putting taste in music and fashion seemed like something he would want to ignore, not encourage.

I thought the music we listened to seriously bothered my mom and dad—but in truth, the thing that really concerned them was that their kids sat down in a basement all day. We didn't do *anything* else. We were achieving a level of chronic laziness that went unsurpassed.

So at dinner, when Nat told them about his idea to start a band, they stared at him over their leftover spaghetti with looks of genuine shock.

"Okay," Mom said, "*if* we could help you find instruments, *if* we let you guys turn the basement into some nightclub, are you going to take it seriously?"

We said that we would.

"No, I mean *seriously*—as in committed," she said. "I mean practicing, lessons, the whole bit. It can't just be like everything else."

We swore that it wouldn't.

If they could help us find some instruments, we would do extra chores, slave labor, whatever—we'd do anything.

"You know," Dad said, "Ronny from Mack & Dave's Pawnshop still owes me some money for doing their books. I could give him a call tomorrow, see what instruments they have."

"That would be *awesome*," I mumbled, while my brain screamed, *Holyshitholyshit!*

For once, maybe something would come easy. Maybe, in a single day, my brother had just kick-started the career of a band that didn't *exist* just hours before. I looked over at him. He was smiling too big to say anything.

* * *

A week passed. Dad didn't mention the pawnshop again. I thought he'd forgotten about the instruments completely.

But the following Saturday, Mom woke me up and told me to get downstairs. I looked out my bedroom window—there was a white moving truck with MACK & DAVE'S stenciled onto the side. I got dressed right away.

Nat was already downstairs, holding the front door open. A couple of guys carried the contents of the truck inside. Their shirts were soiled like they'd been doing heavy lifting since dawn. They glared at us when they passed—*spoiled little fat-asses*—and I was too nervous to ask if I could help.

The last thing they brought inside was a long black case that reminded me of a coffin.

The drum kit had probably been white at some point. But it was old now, and its finish had been timeworn into the yellow hue of stained teeth.

The heads of the drums were stretched to the rims like burnt wax paper. The kit was stacked in pieces around the room. A cymbal the color of a dirty penny leaned against the wall, with a pair of chipped drumsticks on the floor beside it.

"Fuck," I heard Nat say. He was standing over the open case.

"What?"

He pulled out his brand-new, used, bright purple Ibanez bass. I started cracking up.

"Whatever," he said. "I was gonna cover it in stickers anyway."

Dad came down to the basement. He was grinning.

"Well, gentlemen, looks like there is no excuse to be bored anymore."

Mom peeked down a few times too, watching us try to organize the room. The two of them looked happy just to see us doing *something*.

It took over an hour for us to set up the drum kit. I had no idea how to do it, where the drums went, what they were called—I had never even seen a drum kit in person before. All we had to go on was what we'd seen in music videos.

But it was simple enough—snare, tom, floor tom, kick drum—with a cymbal and one broken stand. We covered the stand in duct tape. There was no drum throne, so I used an old painter's stool.

I hit the snare and Mom's hands flew to her ears. My parents didn't come back down to the basement pretty much ever after that.

There was a *Bass for Beginners* book and an electric tuner inside the guitar case. I sat hunched over my stool, watching Nat fiddle with his bass. He was trying to use the tuner.

If the note was out of tune, the tuner flashed red. If it was on the right note, the lights turned green. Nat concentrated, biting his lip as the string stretched tighter over the neck of the bass. I thought it would snap.

But finally, the light turned green.

He plugged the bass into the little amplifier. He strummed an open note. The volume sent sound vibrations up my chest and into my throat. I heard the basement door slam shut.

"You wanna play something?" Nat asked.

"I don't know how to play yet."

"Well, why don't you start by *hitting the drums?*"

I laughed. "Okay, dickhead, cover your ears."

I took the sticks into my hands and hit the snare drum and cymbal. It was *LOUD*—every little addition to the drums seemed to increase the volume a thousandfold. No stereo speakers could ever have matched this sound.

Nat waved his hands for me to stop.

"No, no, dude!" he yelled. "You have to count off!"

"Oh yeah . . ."

He turned his amp up as loud as it would go. I could hear it humming. Nat looked at me and nodded.

I swallowed hard, and my arms tensed. I held the drumsticks up—X—above my head. I nodded back at my brother.

"One!"—*click*—

"Two!"—*click*—

"One! Two! *Onetwothreefour!*"

The room exploded.

THREE

Everyone You'll Never Know

1

Those years were spent underground.

We took the music seriously, just like we promised we would. We picked it up by ear, slowly trying to learn every song in our growing record collection. Other kids came over to jam with us, all of them basically strangers.

For years we struggled at forming a band. Every time we thought we'd found other members, it always seemed to fizzle out after a few rehearsals. It wasn't until we met Brody, standing at the register of Davidson's with the only copy of a Bouncing Souls CD, that things changed.

We'd never met before, because he went to the Catholic school across town. He was tall, with birdlike features. He wore a cabbie hat low on his face. To tell the truth, his spastic energy made me uncomfortable. But he played bass. And he loved punk rock. So fuck it.

Having two bassists was pointless, obviously. So Nat went back to the pawnshop and traded his bass for an electric guitar. He picked power chords up easily, and took to it like a quasi-prodigy.

Two weeks after Nat became an official guitarist, Brody

came over. We learned a cover of "Do What You Want" by Bad Religion. Nat sang it, because no one else would. After playing the same song about a hundred times, I had to admit that we sounded pretty good—we sounded fucking *great*!

The band was on.

We decided to call ourselves DOA—Defiance of Authority. We thought it sounded tough, like a spelled-out middle finger.

We deemed Nat our lead singer by default. The three of us practiced almost every day, learning three or four cover songs a week. It wasn't long before Nat started writing his own material.

Mostly he wrote vague rip-offs of other songs— political shit, love songs, whatever. It was exciting as hell. Whenever I saw him alone, hunched over his guitar scribbling lyrics onto notepads, I felt like I was in a legitimate band.

Not a jam band. Not a cover band. A *band* band—the kind of band that could actually *do something*. The kind of band that could *make it*, whatever that meant.

Except we couldn't get a gig.

We were too loud for open-mic nights. And at fifteen, we weren't old enough to play in the bars. It sucked. We couldn't even play parties, because we were never invited to them. After months of looking for shows, I started thinking that our band might be DOA for real.

It was Paul who had the idea—if no one would book us, we should just put on a concert ourselves. He found two event halls—the VFW and the YWCA—who were willing to rent to minors. Once again by default, Paul became a concert promoter.

The Y was a basically abandoned building on the west end, used for AA meetings and support groups. Paul haggled them down to fifty dollars a night—just $12.50 between the four of us. If we charged five bucks, and ten people came, we could break even. If we got *more* people to come, we agreed to put the extra cash toward having another show.

We started looking for bands to play with. The more bands we could find, the more people might come to the gig. The college was good for a few bands (usually white-dude reggae), and small towns are always good for a few middle-aged heavy metal bands. The guys who begged for change outside of the library told Brody that *they* had a band—an anarchist punk group called Mountain State Militia. They agreed to play the show (if they could borrow our instruments).

Nat made a concert flyer using cutout letters from magazines. I thought it looked more like a ransom note. Dad let us run off copies at his office—we made a hundred. The black ink was hot to the touch.

We skated all around town with the flyers. We taped them up on poles and storefront windows, in bathrooms and on stop signs. Davidson's put one on their door. The only place in town that we *didn't* put up flyers was school—if the show sucked, I didn't want anyone there to see it.

* * *

Nat and I showed up to the YWCA early, so no one would see our parents drop us off. We helped Paul move all the folding chairs into a corner, while Brody set up the PA on the small stage. The other bands arrived around six, and soon it was almost time for the show to start.

I can remember standing in the corner, watching people file in as Paul worked the door. Everyone looked at least ten years older than me. A few seemed wasted. I saw tattoos of roses and faded barbed wire. One guy wore a cutoff Misfits shirt down past his knees. A group of crusty punks showed up out of nowhere, all wearing camo and black. Paul told me later that they smelled like old dog food, and paid the cover in change.

Twenty-two people showed up for that show.

Twenty-two people saw a handmade poster for a punk rock concert in an abandoned YWCA and *came*! It was fucking amazing—all these semi-punks and loners had been living in my town, and before that night I hadn't even known it.

When the first band started, no one was sure what to do. No bands ever came through Huntington, and none of us were used to being at concerts. All we could do was imitate what we saw in videos and magazines. A couple guys headbanged, and one tried (unsuccessfully) to start a mosh pit.

But by the time Defiance of Authority went on, the crowd was all warmed up. We played mostly cover songs, and snuck the few originals that Nat had written into the set. Playing to an audience was so different from jamming in the basement. I could barely focus on what I was doing.

The crowd finally started moshing a little, and when we played our Bad Religion cover, the guys who were dancing ended up on the stage. They ran into each other, pushing and spitting at us, bumping into our equipment. It was one of the best nights of my life.

*   *   *

And so that was that.

Nat kept writing songs. Paul kept putting on shows—and the crowds kept growing. Some kids came to check out the music. Most just came for something to do. But for those of us who considered ourselves punk rockers, the chance to meet other like-minded losers was huge.

A few others started putting on their own shows. A lot of kids decided to form bands of their own. Soon there was a show at least every two weeks. Time was now measured by concerts.

My brother soon turned from a "singer" into a front man. He wanted to *look* like a lead singer—he dyed his hair jet-black, contorting it into a pathetic replica of a Social Distortion pompadour. Onstage he would wear only black.

By the time we entered high school, we both needed glasses. I ended up with a pair of thick-rimmed black frames that made my eyes look huge. Nat refused to wear any. He said it would "fuck up his stage presence." He said he'd rather go blind.

When we were sixteen, Nat convinced me to bleach my hair from blond to white. He thought it would help us stand out more onstage. I ended up with a burnt scalp and hair the color of unhealthy piss. I dug it. I spent a half hour each morning using gobs of glue to spike it into brutally sharp points.

Nat was right—for the first time, we weren't identical. You'd never be able to tell we were twins, unless you saw us together.

And we were always together.

* * *

By the time I was seventeen, we were pulling in about a hundred kids a show. We were *sure* we could get a big-time record deal now—we just weren't sure how to make it happen.

We recorded demo tape after demo tape of our original material. I mailed copies out to Epitaph Records, Nitro Records, Lookout! Records, Fat Wreck Chords—all the record labels that specialized in punk bands.

I'm still waiting to hear back from them.

In terms of business, it was Brody who really started guiding the band. He found countless books on the music business—touring, management, promotion. After reading a few, he realized some contained lists of contacts.

So—like my brother with his liner notes—Brody plowed through each book, making spreadsheets of label addresses, booking agencies, tour promoters, phone numbers, e-mails, and contacts. He was sure that it was common sense, not songwriting, that would finally score us a record deal.

His latest plan was to get us on the Warped Tour.

Magazine ads for the past five Warped Tours were taped

on the walls of our basement—Pennywise, Social D, Sublime, Bad Religion, FEAR, Descendents—*all* of our favorite bands went on this tour! It was like a punk rock circus, all these awesome bands in one place—every summer, when the tour kicked off, I ached to get to go to a show. But we lived in West Virginia. No tours ever passed through.

In the back of the book *Everyone You'll Never Know: An Insider's Guide Through the Music Biz*, Brody hit the fucking jackpot—he found the contact information for Kevin Lyman, the organizer of the tour.

So he mailed him our latest demo and a handwritten letter of adoration. Brody was sure it would butter him up enough to put Defiance of Authority on the tour.

If we could get on Warped, we could get a record deal. When record-label fat cats came to see the bands on their rosters, we would be waiting. We'd beg, we'd plead, we wouldn't let them leave until they watched us play.

Brody was certain his new plan would work.

I had faith in the plan too—why wouldn't I? It was nice to imagine leaving our town, nice to imagine the band having a shot at the big time. It was nice to have a plan.

So, at seventeen—while school got harder, the girls got scarier, and adulthood loomed on the horizon—I didn't pay anything much mind. All that shit seemed secondary to me now.

School was nothing but a waiting room.

2

Nat and I shared a 1986 Ford Astrovan named Sheena. Her windows were tinted, and her left brake light was cracked. She was painted the color of pond scum. We'd covered her backside in stickers and hung dice from the rearview mirror. There was a tape deck that worked okay, and the previous owner had installed a CD player. But her upholstery—covered in stains and cigarette burns—showed her age.

Other kids might have been embarrassed to drive an old van, but not us. We fucking loved it. Because we only thought of Sheena in her official capacity—*tour van*.

Of course, we had no tours to go on. But that wasn't the point.

Touring was *eventual*—if we didn't get on the Warped Tour, something else would come along. Maybe one of our demo tapes would finally be heard, and we'd score some huge record deal—it didn't matter how we got the record deal; we'd get to go on tour and promote the record. So having a van put us ahead of the curve—when the future came calling, we would be ready.

* * *

While we waited for Epitaph Records to track us down, we mostly used the tour van to drive to school. Paul rode with us every morning, although he cared about school even less than me. By eleventh grade, he didn't even bring his books.

Huntington High sat on a steep hill outside of town. Only one road led to the school, and each morning we took our place in the clogged line of buses and muddy pickups. On top of the hill was a flagpole where the Christian kids did a morning prayer. I ignored them on my way into the building.

The walls were lined with massive trophy cases, which were mostly a shrine to then current sports heroes. I often saw them smiling at themselves through the dirty glass. Our same little gang stood together beneath the stairwell.

When the first bell rang it meant I had to leave my friends. I strolled down the hallway alone, into the fuck-off that defined my high school existence.

I sat in the back singing songs, undressing girls, and watching music videos all in my head—but mostly, I thought about my band.

I wrote setlists for imaginary tours, I chose outfits to wear onstage, I dreamed up countless album covers—anything not to focus on how slow the minute hand moved.

* * *

If there wasn't a punk show going on, we spent Saturday nights just driving around. Nat, Paul, and I—sometimes more, never less—would just get into the van, crank the stereo, and go.

We would cruise all around the town—past the park and its empty benches, past the public pool now drained and abandoned. We took the winding hill up Washington Boulevard, where the houses grew larger by the block. On the other side of the hill, the houses got small again. Drunken railroad workers spilt out of dive bars, onto the sidewalks. From there, we drove into downtown, past rows and rows of boarded-up storefronts.

We always ended up at the river.

We parked past the flood wall, which blocked out the

few lights still burning behind us. We'd sit in the van with our seat belts off, barely speaking. The moon was bright on the river, floating eternally downstream.

After we had driven the entire town, there was nothing left to do but circle back. Back to the east end, or maybe to the west. We didn't care where we ended up. There was no destination. We covered ground aimlessly, like animals pacing in a cage.

3

I tried to talk to the girls in my class. The attempts were pathetically executed. Nat said that I was overly complimentary; I focused on small things—nail polish, perfume—stuff I figured their boyfriends never noticed.

Sometimes the girls were nice enough to let me ramble on, until they could break away from the conversation politely. But I knew they didn't take me seriously—fuck, how could they? Everything I said came off as grossly innocent.

So mainly, I just watched them.

Not like a creep or anything—I just mean that I *admired* them.

A lot.

I admired the way they brushed their hair behind their ears as they smiled, and the sound of their laughter down the halls. I was amazed how these creatures seemed so unaware of their sex—their breasts, their curves, all perfect by existence alone. I memorized the quarter-inch gaps between the bottoms of their shirts and the tops of their pants.

I focused like my glasses gave me X-ray eyes.

I stood in the hallways, and I leaned on the walls. I watched girl after girl after girl after girl after girl after girl after girl after girl after girl after girl after girl after girl.

I felt lucky just to be that close.

FOUR

Shitsville, USA

1

Ali Wilhelm was in the top tier of girls who passed me in the hallway each morning. She was one of the best-looking chicks in the whole fucking school. Guys wasted their Friday nights at football games just so they could watch her clap and bounce with the rest of the cheerleading squad. She had long black hair she wore straight down her shoulders, the way an Indian princess or metalhead might. Her skin was gold, no matter the season.

I'd see her with her boyfriends in the parking lot after school—always jocks and good-looking and older. The yearbook committee even voted her "Best Smile" every year—I mean, this chick was award-winning.

She lived up on Washington Boulevard, like all her friends. They were all cheerleaders. They were all loaded. They were all gorgeous. And they all ignored me.

Except for Mandy, Ali's best friend.

Mandy was big and blond, with tits so huge that they circled from bad to good, then back to bad again. She was the ugliest of the pretty girls, but she refused to be overshadowed by her cheerleader friends. She got her attention by being the loudest person in the room. Any room.

The two of them walked through school together every morning.

That morning, I was in the hallway doing my thing. I could hear Mandy's bellow before the two of them were ever in sight. When Mandy and Ali rounded the corner, they were both laughing. *They must be stoned,* I thought. *No one laughs that fucking hard this early.*

I scoped out Ali as she walked. I watched her body move—left foot, right foot, left hip, right hip, right breast, left breast—everything pulsed to some forbidden beat that my eyes couldn't quite stay in time with. Watching. Leching. Ogling. I couldn't help it. Her voodoo strut hypnotized me.

"Hey!" Mandy yelled my way.

Fuck. I was busted. *Shit.* I was a complete creep.

I tried to look away, but they were already walking toward me.

"Hi," I mumbled. It was the closest I'd ever stood to either of them.

Ali—*jesusfuckingchrist, man.* She was even prettier up close.

And she had freckles—she was *covered* in freckles. How had I never noticed? They made intricate patterns under her eyes. They ran down her neckline, speckling the bones above her breasts before they disappeared down her shirt.

I tried not to stare, kind of.

"You're Nat's brother, right?" Mandy asked.

"We're twins."

"Um, ya think? No shit." She rolled her eyes and smiled.

"I love Nat," Ali said. Her voice was raspier than I'd expected. "He's so funny! We have seventh period together."

"Nat's *way* hotter," Mandy said. "I like that all-black look." She looked back at me. "What's his deal? He dating anyone?"

A few months before, Nat had met a chick named Ashley at one of our shows. She was a quiet, mousy thing who'd just started her first semester at college. She was too shy to talk to me or Paul—but she'd talk to him. Lately, the two of them had been spending a lot of time together.

"I mean, he kinda has a girlfriend."

"Well shit," she yelled. "Let me guess, one of those Marilyn Manson–looking bitches?"

"Yeah. Pretty much."

"*Gross.* Ugh. Well, you tell your brother to come talk to me when he wants a *real* girl—tell him that just 'cause I don't look like Dracula, it doesn't mean I can't suck! Ha!"

"Oh my God," Ali said, slapping Mandy on the arm.

We shared a look—only for a second—and then our eyes fell to the floor.

"I'll let him know," I said.

"Fuck, yes, you will," Mandy said. She flashed another all-teeth grin, and then started walking.

Ali lingered behind, barely. I had to say *something* to her.

"I . . . I dig your nail polish," I stammered.

Idiot! I didn't even know if she was wearing nail polish. It just came out.

She lifted up her hand—her nails were a chipped apple green. She smiled. She didn't reply, but she smiled that smile.

And then she was gone.

———

In class, I dreamed of her freckles. I imagined the ones on her neck, glowing with the rhythm of her breath—dim, rising easy, and then glowing again, lit up like constellations in my young, lonely mind.

2

I decided to invite Ali to our show on Saturday.

Normally, I wouldn't have dared. Some people at school vaguely knew I was in a band, but that was it. No one had actually *heard* us—if someone came and thought we sucked, I imagined I'd be getting picked on even worse than we did back in junior high.

But she smiled at me—that must mean something.

So the next morning, I spiked my hair extra spiky. I wore my red button-up shirt—it had a collar, so I thought she would like it. Before I went downstairs, I shoved a show flyer into my pocket.

I leaned against the same locker at school. Hands in my pockets—*James Dean cool.*

Mandy walked by with a group of boys, but no Ali. The final bell rang, and classroom doors began to shut. The hall emptied. I just stood there.

I counted the seconds. *Is it creepy to wait here like this?* I wondered. I heard my brother's voice inside my head, saying, *If you have to ask, then it is.*

I sighed. Forget it.

I grabbed my backpack and started walking to class—but then she appeared, stumbling quickly down the middle of the hall. Her hair was a mess. She wore the same clothes as the day before.

Rumors popped in my mind—all the popular kids are druggies, train wrecks. *Nah,* not her. People like me just said that sorta stuff because we were jealous. I waved toward her, but she was staring straight down.

"*Yo,* Ali!"

She looked up. "Oh . . . hey."

Even without makeup, even in the soiled clothes, I couldn't imagine this girl as a train wreck—Mandy, maybe, but not her. Not a girl like this. Her eyes were clear, like little black pebbles. I dismissed the gossip as bullshit.

"Long night?" I asked.

"Uggghh, yeah. I was busy all night."

"Me too," I lied. "I'm glad I ran into you, though. I wanted to . . ." I fumbled in my pocket for the flyer.

My fingers were too sweaty to grip it. My hand got twisted inside my pocket. I yanked at it. She looked at my pants.

Finally, I yanked out the flyer and *shoved* it into her chest.

". . . I wanted to give you that," I finished. I grinned nervously.

My sweaty hand had left the flyer looking like a used napkin. Ali straightened it out on her jeans.

"It's a flyer for our show this weekend."

"No way!" she said, skimming it. "Which band is yours?"

"Defiance of Authority."

"Ha. I mean, *cool*. I keep telling Nat I wanna see y'all play. I don't think he believes me."

"Nat never believes anyone about anything."

"Saturday? Hmmm, well—maybe I need to come and prove him wrong."

I nodded. "Yeah, maybe you should."

"Maybe I will."

"Yeah?"

"Yep."

"Well, right on."

I shrugged apathetically. Ali folded the flyer and stuck it in her back pocket.

"I gotta go," she said. "This semester just started, and I've already been late about ten times."

I flashed the peace sign—*V* for fucking victory. I leaned back against the locker and watched her go.

James Dean cool.

3

By the time dark came, the lot beside the YWCA was full. Used cars were parked crookedly, covered in stickers and beat to shit. Punks leaned against them, huddled together breathing blue smoke into the cold. A few drank from paper bags. The streetlights on the corner made them look like shadows.

Once the opening band was set up, Paul popped the door and people filed through it. I saw Egor come in, even more metal now dangling from his face. I saw a couple tattoos but no freckles. I saw druggies walk by, but I didn't see Ali.

Even if Ali didn't show up, watching the crowd walk

through the door wasn't without pleasure. It was nice to see the way shoulders eased as people came inside. I knew it had little to do with the cold—these shows were our break from "normal" life, a recharge from the exhausting pressures of existence. The shows were a bloodletting.

The shows were five bucks at the door.

*　*　*

The third band was finishing their set. The crowd had doubled in size by now, and the room was getting packed. We were on next. Ali still hadn't shown.

She had probably never actually planned on coming in the first place. *Fuck it.* I gave up on watching the door.

Someone tugged at my arm—it was Paul.

"Yo man—y'all are on," he said.

I hadn't even noticed that the music had stopped.

I joined Nat and Brody in the corner, and we lugged our gear up to the stage. I arranged my drums exactly as I did at practice, and made sure my cymbal stands were tightened tight. Nat taped his guitar cables to the floor. Brody tuned his bass, tugging at the shoulder strap to make sure it would hold.

We went out of our way to avoid any fuckups.

The crowd stayed close to the stage, talking amongst themselves. They didn't walk outside the way they did when the other bands set up. For us, they waited.

Nat turned his back to the crowd and looked at me. He nodded, I nodded back—it was time.

He pointed his guitar toward the speaker of his amp,

twisting his volume knob to create feedback. I raised my sticks into the air, but Nat shook his head—*not yet.*

The squeal of the amp grew louder. The crowd covered their ears, cursing.

Nat nodded—*now.*

"One!"—*click*—

"Two!"—*click*—

"One! Two! *Onetwothreefour!*"

Nat and Brody both jumped into the air, landing on beat with the first cymbal crash. Nat pounded the strings of his guitar.

"Let's GO!" Brody yelled into the mic.

The crowd yelled back.

We opened with a song called "Watch You Fall," because it was the fastest one we had. Not that it really made a difference—when we played live, *every* song became the fastest song. No matter how much I practiced, the second I was in front of an audience I pounded through each song at warp speed. I couldn't help it—I felt the energy of the room, and the tension in my arms as my sticks *hit, hit, hit, hit*—damn, man!

It was exciting. If that meant I played a little too fast—screw it.

Traditionally, the band follows the drummer. But in our band, I followed Nat—completely zoning out the rest of the stage. So no matter if we played sloppy or tight, the two of us were always in time with each other.

After the third song ended we held for applause.

This was the part of the set where Nat fucked around with the crowd. I don't remember what he said—all that

I remember is hearing that laugh. That *bellow*—heavy, coming back at us.

I froze.

She—*they*—were standing right there. Ali and Mandy, second row, stage left. They both waved.

I was instantly nervous. My arms turned to rubber. I looked down, over, up—anywhere but back toward the crowd.

Nat nodded at me, and I counted us into the next song. I got through the first verse okay—but I messed up two drum fills, and at the end of the song I dropped a stick. . . . I just couldn't concentrate. Seeing Ali caught me way off guard.

Performing for a crowd and performing for a girl are completely different things—a guy needs time to mentally prepare for that shit, you know?

Now I was running on autopilot, hoping enough muscle memory would kick in to get me through the rest of the set. I didn't once look back toward her.

Five songs later, the show was mercifully over.

It's always amazed me how fast a crowd breaks up at the end of a concert. All these people sing and dance together—but the second the music ends, they file toward their cars like polite strangers. I left my kit and pushed against the moving crowd, heading quickly for the back of the building.

I knew Nat and Brody were going to bitch me out for playing so bad, and I was already humiliated enough. All I wanted to do now was escape.

I moved past the bathrooms and into the hall, toward

the back door. I'd wait outside while the room cleared out. I didn't want to see anyone—Ali and Mandy especially—or hear any half-assed "good show" comments.

I grabbed the door handle—it was cold. Good. That's what I needed—to cool down, catch my breath, and hide.

"Good show," a voice I couldn't yet connect to a body said.

I gritted my teeth. I was sitting on the ground with my head against the wall. My wet T-shirt was frozen to my body. I looked up.

It was Ali. She was alone too, hugging herself from the wind. A cigarette dangled between her fingers.

"Thanks," I said, embarrassed. I stood up and shoved my hands in my pockets. "I didn't really think you'd come."

She took a drag from her cigarette. I could feel her look me over. My fucking *goose bumps* got goose bumps.

"I didn't think I would either. Mandy's in charge of driving tonight—I ended up having to tell her that Nat had a thing for her just to get her fat ass to come down."

I laughed. We moved closer to each other without realizing it.

"But you guys were, like, *good!*" she said.

"Ha—don't sound so shocked."

"I didn't mean it like that. Okay, well maybe I did. I knew you'd be *good*, I just didn't know that I would, like, *like* it!"

"Well, thanks," I said. "I know this scene can seem a little *odd*."

Ali exhaled.

"So, where's Mandy," I asked, trying not to cough. "Hunting down my bro?"

"Nah, in the car. She said she was gonna warm it up while I smoked, but I just *know* that bitch is snorting up all the Purple Footballs we bought."

"Lame," I said, not knowing what a Purple Football even was. Later, when my world became one large medicine cabinet, I learned it was a tag for Xanax, the wonder drug. "What are y'all doing for the rest of the night?"

"Adam Goldstein's having a party. So the usual."

Everyone knew Adam's house. It was the biggest one in town, at the very top of Washington Boulevard. I'd never been invited to one of his parties, but many Saturday nights I saw the lights burning as we drove by—saw silhouettes stumbling in the dark outside, teens doubling as drunken lawn art. I tried not to imagine her as part of the landscaping.

"Sweet," I said.

She shrugged. "It's whatever."

She flicked her cigarette into the dark.

"Looks like you're done with your smoke."

"Looks like it."

We locked eyes—just for a second. She broke her gaze first and dug through the small purse hanging from her shoulder.

"So," she said, "you want to hang out with me again sometime, or what?"

"YEAH!"—I cleared my throat—"I mean, sure. That'd be cool."

She grinned, pulled a pen from her purse, and popped the cap with her teeth.

"Gimme," she said, grabbing my hand.

She led me to where the light from the door made the blacktop shine. I could see her hand—her nails were freshly painted black. The tip of her pen dug into my clammy palm. She tattooed her phone number into my skin.

634-3433

"Call me, drummer boy," she said. She put the pen back into her purse, and then she disappeared.

I heard a car door open. I heard it slam shut.

I stood in the cold alone. I held my hand up to the sky, inspecting it in that sliver of light. I traced the dark blue lines that she'd put on my palm. I followed each one. I read my future.

4

I woke up thinking in dial tones.

I looked at my hand—it was nothing but a blue smear. I'd rubbed most of Ali's number off during the night.

I flew out of bed, running her number through my memory while I searched for a pen. *SIXTHREEFOUR-THREEFOURTHREETHREE!* I wrote her number down on the face of my small desk and let out a sigh of relief.

I got back in bed and shut my eyes.

The number kept playing in my head. I heard it in different patterns and melodies—even the tempos changed. But the lyrics were always the same—*sixthree four three four threethree*—my dial was tuned to the *Wilhelm Power Hour*, only on 634.3433 FM—*your station for all Ali, all the time.*

* * *

Nat was ignoring me. He was still pissed that I'd blown our show. Which sucked, because I really needed his advice.

I mean, he *had* a girlfriend—but at seventeen, I still had almost zero experience with chicks. I wasn't sure how I'd gotten Ali's attention in the first place, but the fact that I hadn't lost it yet was a small miracle. One misstep could ruin the whole thing.

So I needed advice—how had he gotten Ashley to like him? What made her take him so seriously?

But unless I was telling him I'd signed up for drum lessons, Nat had no interest in talking to me. I was on my own.

So I thought about him and Ashley, trying to remember little things that happened when they first started hanging out. The memory that stuck out the clearest was when Ashley made him a mixtape, before she went home over Christmas break.

Now, all our friends made mixtapes—skating mixes, Halloween mixes, best-of mixes—so I never thought it was a big deal. But when she made Nat one, I could tell it was something different.

Maybe it was the order of the songs, or maybe it was the lyrics. Maybe it was the little hearts Ashley drew on the label. Whatever made it special, Nat was *obsessed* with that tape. He treated it like a coded message, a prized possession, a sacred thing.

There must be something to that, right?

I knocked on the door of Nat's bedroom.

"What?" he yelled through the door.

"Hey, dude. I know I fucked up the show super bad. And I know you don't wanna talk to me. All I want to know is, do you have any blank tapes?"

*   *   *

I knelt before the stereo.

It was well past midnight. Tapes and CDs were freed from their jewel cases and spread all around me. Near them was the cellophane wrap of the fresh, untouched cassette. I plugged in a set of headphones so I wouldn't wake anyone up.

I'd been working on her tape for hours. It was hard picking songs—there are endless numbers of love songs, even in punk rock, but a tape full of love songs was too predictable. I wanted this tape to be full of songs that Ali might actually *like*.

I didn't want to use anything too cheesy or depressing (none of Nat and Ashley's slit-your-wrist-type emo shit). I didn't want to seem too forward, but I needed my intentions to be unmistakable. Otherwise, even if Ali and I started hanging out, I was likely to fumble my way into the friend zone.

Making this tape was a chance to prove myself, to show off my *true* talent—not playing music, but feeling it. Because at the end of the day, I never considered myself anything more than a fan.

I made sure the tape was rewound. I pressed the play and record buttons with all my might:

DIE YOUNG WITH ME

Ali's Mix

SIDE A

1. Nada Surf—"Popular"
2. Descendents—"This Place"
3. Blink-182—"Untitled"
4. Rancid—"She's Automatic"
5. Sublime—"Smoke Two Joints"
6. Black Flag—"Wasted"
7. Dead Milkmen—"Punk Rock Girl"
8. The Misfits—"Skulls"
9. The Humpers—"Mutate with Me"

SIDE B

1. The Ataris—"Your Boyfriend Sucks"
2. Bad Religion—"21st Century (Digital Boy)"
3. Descendents—"I'm the One"
4. Social Distortion—"When She Begins"
5. Everclear—"Sparkle and Fade"
6. Screeching Weasel—"Hey Suburbia"
7. Face to Face—"Ordinary"
8. Lagwagon—"Brown Eyed Girl"
9. The Ramones—"I Want You Around"

Each song wasn't my favorite, but every song had a place. I tried not to overdo the love songs. I spaced the whiny songs between heavier ones. I added a couple of tracks about feeling like an outcast. I even added a few songs about doing drugs, just to be safe. I wanted a lyric, a hook, *something* to grab her, the same way that it had grabbed me. I knew that it wasn't a perfect group of songs, but I hoped it was perfect for her.

I wrote *Ali's Mix* on the label.

5

It took until Tuesday to muster the balls that were needed to give her the tape. She seemed excited—but as the days went on, she never mentioned it again.

It took a whole other week to finally get a date with her—on a Thursday night. She said that her weekends were all booked up.

She was hard to read or I was bad at reading. Either way, she hadn't distanced herself from me yet. We met every morning at the lockers, there in front of my class. Ali stood a little closer to me now, and a little was all that I needed.

It was close enough for me to feel the heat coming off her body. It was close enough for me to smell her hair— the mixed aroma of cigarette smoke and apricot shampoo.

* * *

I was painfully nervous about the date. I'd only been on one other date in my life, and it was a total fucking disaster.

The girl's name was Danielle Maraquin. She had just transferred into our eighth-grade class from Wayne

County. She was ethnic looking in a nondescript way—her skin was dark, her arms were covered in black hair. One of her front teeth was oddly missing.

But Danielle already had tits. And her jeans were tight. And she liked me—sort of. Not a lot, but enough to let me take her to the movies.

We met at the theater, where she chose some Ethan Hawke flick I didn't want to see. But I bought our tickets and a large popcorn.

She wanted to sit in the very back row. She knew that I was nervous. She even laughed about it. But then the previews started up, and we sat in silence.

About an hour into the movie, she asked if I wanted to kiss her.

I said yes.

Danielle ran her hand down my cheek. I turned my face toward her. Sparks lit through my legs and guts. The colors of the movie reflected in her eyes. She looked almost beautiful in the darkness, her missing tooth now only a shadow in the projector's flickering dreamglow.

She led me toward her lips. I leaned in and closed my eyes. My lips puckered, searching for hers.

And then she burped—right in my goddamn face.

The word *burp* doesn't begin to describe this disgusting, malicious popcorn belch. Worst of all, my surprise caused me to inhale—sucking her buttery stomach acid in through my lips.

"Don't you want to kiss me?" she cackled through her insane jack-o'-lantern smile.

She *grabbed* my face and jammed her lips onto mine. I felt the wet nub of her tongue dart in and out of my mouth, shooting from side to side as though it were locked in a trunk.

I couldn't shake the memory of it. I mean, I didn't know much about Ali, but I knew that at the very least, she had all her teeth. I was so out of my depth that it was hard to breathe. *Can I hold her hand? Can I kiss her? Can I should I could I dammit fuck shitshitfuckshit!* I didn't know what the hell I was doing.

I'd been sitting in Ali's driveway for fifteen minutes, agonizing over whether I should even go through with it. Maybe I should save us both the trouble and bail.

I put on music to clear my head.

I searched around for something good. I'd borrowed Mom's car for the date, because I feared a van might make a kidnappy first impression. But the only CDs she had were Rod Stewart and Mary Chapin Carpenter. So I flipped on the radio.

It was on 97.9 Golden Oldies—man, I hadn't listened to that station since I was little. Dad used to blast it—*mood music*, he always said.

"Cupid" by Sam Cooke was playing. I turned it up.

*I know between the two of us her heart we can steal
Help me, if you will . . .*

I took it as a sign, from Cupid himself, or some black, well-dressed rock 'n' roll God in the sky—it had to be. I mean, Sam Cooke would never let inexperience stand in the way of a fine-ass girl like Ali, would he? Not a chance.

"Fuck it," I said out loud.

I checked my look in the rearview, popped in some gum, sucked in my gut, and strutted up to her door.

* * *

Ali's older sister Liz answered. She was a year ahead of us, one of the senior girls who I was scared to even look at. Liz was taller than Ali, and her hair was the almost-red of burning leaves—but otherwise, the two of them looked nearly identical.

"Hi Roooobbb!" she said. She was smiling Ali's smile.

Then she hugged me—*tight*.

My hello got trapped between her cleavage. I tried not to drool, or accidentally lick anything. She finally let go and held me at arm's length, looking me up and down.

"I've heard a lot about you," she said.

"That's a scary thought."

"Is that him?" a voice yelled from the stairs behind her.

"Yes, Mom, Jesus!" Liz yelled back.

A squat woman came charging down the stairs like a boulder. She looked like she'd spent the entire 1980s inside a tanning bed.

"I *told* you not to use the Lord's name in vain, dammit," she snapped. Then she looked at me. "So you're the musician?"

I nodded.

"You know who Frankie Valli is?"

"Sure," I said.

She smiled. "Where I grew up, Frankie was bigga than Elvis. He was an *angel*. I lived right near his house and when my friends and I would walk by, he'd come right out on the porch, and—"

"*Mom*," Ali yelled, rushing down the stairs, "*please* shut up."

She pushed through my welcoming committee and moved right past me. She wore tight gray pants and a red flannel peacoat. Her lips looked darker.

"We're leaving—*now*," she said. "Quit bugging him. Come on, Rob."

"Yes, ma'am," I said.

The mom and sister laughed.

"*Byeeeee,*" they sang, mockingly sweet.

I followed Ali to the car. I opened the door for her.

Once she got inside, she leaned back and took a deep breath.

"Sorry," she said. "They always do that. It drives me fucking crazy." She turned to me. "Can we go? I have another sister, three brothers, and a dad who'll be coming down any second if we don't leave."

"Shit," I said. "Yeah . . . don't worry—your getaway driver is here."

I turned over the engine.

The radio jolted alive. The McCoys were in the middle of "Hang On, Sloopy." *Hang on,* I thought to myself. I shifted into reverse, gunning the car down her driveway backward as gravel crunched beneath us. I cut the tires at the edge of the road so hard that they squealed. Dust blew around us.

"My hero." Ali laughed.

She turned the radio louder as we drove into the dark.

* * *

We sat in a back booth at Chili Willi's Mexican Cantina. The place was so empty, it seemed like we had the whole restaurant to ourselves.

As far as I could tell, the night was going okay. Ali was laughing at my jokes, and I'd managed to keep her talking, but now that we'd finished our burritos, the conversation started to lag.

I was getting nervous, and drummed on the table awkwardly as I waited on the check. The opening riff to "Blaze of Glory" sounded from the radio at the bar.

"I love this song," Ali said.

"Really?"

"Uh, duh. Mom's from Jersey—she forced Bon Jovi on us."

I thought of that day Nat burnt our Bon Jovi albums, in his alleyway sacrifice to the punk rock gods.

"I dig Jovi too," I said.

"Really? I thought they might be too *normal* for you."

I shook my head. "No way—I like all different types of music."

"Yeah? So what's the best Bon Jovi song?"

Luckily, it didn't matter how much I loved or hated a band, record, or song—when it came to music, my memory was on point.

"Probably 'I'll Be There for You.'"

"Not 'Livin' on a Prayer'?"

I shrugged. "Isn't that one a little normal?"

Ali smiled. "Okay, 'Bad Medicine.'"

"I like 'Always.'"

She threw a tortilla chip at me. "You pussy. Maybe you should listen to 'Let It Rock' or something."

"What about 'Wild in the Streets'?"

"I like 'Bed of Roses,' " she said.

"Jesus, and *I'm* the pussy? Shit! 'Never Say Goodbye' is a better slow jam than that."

Ali didn't answer me. Our waiter came back with my change.

"I'm sorry. Did I say something dumb?"

"No, you're fine. It's just, that song makes me sad. It's like—*we* are graduating in a year and a half. *Then* what? Do we end up like the people in that song? Wishing we were in high school forever? It's just depressing."

She took a sip of her Diet Coke.

"I never thought about it like that." I hadn't.

I leaned in closer. "It's cool you heard all that in the lyrics. Most people don't ever pay attention to what songs are trying to say, even if it's one of their favorites. No one ever cares."

Ali just shrugged. She stood up and put on her coat.

"Okay," she said, "one last good Jovi song before we leave—'Lay Your Hands on Me.' " She winked.

She fucking *winked*.

I opened my mouth to reply, but there was no point— the song was over now, the bar radio was playing the Eagles. Our moment was gone.

* * *

She asked if I'd swing by the park before I drove her home.

Ritter Park was halfway between my house and hers. It had tennis courts and a rose garden, muddy hiking trails and a playground, but the park itself was barren. Nothing but an occasional pine tree or pile of dogshit occupied the otherwise empty stretch of green.

When she asked me to take her there, I wondered if she really did want me to lay my hands on her. I ran five red lights on my way to that fucking park, but as we got closer, Ali said that she only needed to pick something up.

"What's there to pick up in a park, in the middle of the night?"

"Uh, weed, pills. You know—drugs," she said, shaking her head.

I laughed nervously.

"Is that okay?" She touched my arm. "I thought you said you were my getaway driver."

"Uh noyeah yep yeahyeah it's totallyfinetotallycool," I sputtered.

I ran another red light.

The park was empty. Ali directed me to the back of the lot beside the playground. It was empty too.

Less than a minute after we parked, a black sedan pulled in slooooooowly. It stopped at the opposite end of the lot. No one got out.

My eyes darted in all directions. I was ready to floor it at any second.

"Be right back," she said cheerfully.

She walked across the lot. A black window rolled down, and a black arm reached out as Ali's reached in. She stuffed her hand into her pocket and walked in my direction. The sedan pulled out of the lot with its head-lights off.

When she rapped on my window I jumped, and my

hand hit the horn. She started cracking up. I laughed too, relieved that the deal was done. I cracked the window.

"All good?"

"Yep," she said.

She pulled her cigarettes from her other pocket. She put one between her lips and leaned in toward my window as she lit it. She stepped back and blew smoke into heaven.

"Feel like keeping me company while I smoke this?"

"You know it," I said.

We walked through the deserted playground, past the rusty swings and the slide. Somewhere near the sandbox, she let me hold her hand. Beyond it was a bench swing that faced outward, toward the rest of the park.

We sat down on the cold wood.

We rocked slowly back and forth, our toes scraping the ground. Ali smoked her cigarette. We held hands. We didn't talk.

The park stretched into the darkness, until the shaded green landscape joined with the night and the stars. I couldn't see the houses and I couldn't see the street. There were no cars. All was quiet. We were staring out at a secret ocean.

"You don't get high, do you?" she asked.

I shook my head.

"How come?"

"I dunno, really. I just don't. I don't drink either—I mean, I don't care if *you* do—I'm trying to stay focused on my band, and I get scared that doin' that shit would cloud my mind."

"Well, yeah—that's the whole point," she said.

"Ha, right. I guess it is."

She tossed away her butt and immediately took out another cigarette. I held my hand over her lighter until the flame caught.

"It helps me with my anxiety," she said, "ya know? Helps me get outta my own head."

"Yeah," I said, looking into the dark, "I gave up on getting out of my head. At this point I just focus on getting out of this town."

"Yeah?"

I nodded. "*Totally*—shit, at least there'd be some good concerts."

"What do you *mean*? I just saw a great show! Some punk band, I wish I could remember the name, but they did have this really cute drummer."

"Hm. Who knows."

I smiled inside. We sat and rocked a little longer.

"Y'all really are awesome, Rob. You guys will get famous, I bet."

"Nah, not here, at least."

"You don't know that," she said.

"Yeah—I really do. No bands even tour through here, unless you count stopping for gas. Every record company is pretty much in LA or New York."

"So what are you gonna do?"

I shrugged. "Tour to LA or New York, I guess. Try to get their attention."

"You just better not forget about your number one fan when you're all famous, drummer boy."

"Hey. You might be a lot of things, but forgettable isn't one of them."

She tucked her head underneath my arm.

"Do you really think Huntington is that bad?" she asked.

"What—you mean Shitsville, USA? Um, yes."

She laughed. "Shitsville. That's good. I always call it 'The Great American Pit Stop.' "

"Sounds about right."

"I dunno. I joke about it a lot, but I don't think it's so terrible."

"Easy for you to say," I mumbled. "Life looks a lot different at the cool kids' table."

Ali winced. Her hand slipped away from mine.

Fuck! Moron!

"Oh man . . . shit, Ali . . . I didn't mean anything by that," I pleaded. "Sorry . . . shit, *seriously*—I'm sorry . . ."

"You don't think I'm already used to hearing that? Rich bitch, cheerleader cunt—whatever. Like, there's no chance that *maybe* things aren't so great for me here either? Maybe things *suck* for me . . . but so what, right? No one cares. Forget it, I'm used to it."

I took her hand back. "Come on. That isn't true. *I care*—seriously."

She stared at the ground and pushed the swing faster.

"What do your parents do?" she finally said.

"My dad's a CPA and teaches at the college. My mom works at the refinery, over in Ashland. What about yours?"

"Nothing," she said. "Dad works—*worked*—for the lottery, but he lost his job a few months ago. His boss got indicted for embezzlement, or something. They fired my dad too, even though he had no idea."

"Holy shit."

"He got royally fucked. It's just . . . it's all really fucked up. Like—*fuck*—you know what I mean?"

I forced a smile. "Yeah, but come on—your dad must be *super* smart if he worked for the lotto. Right? He'll get a new gig soon."

"Rob, you don't get it."

"No, I guess not," I said.

"You know the worst part? My friends are already making plans for college—UK, OSU—it's *all* they fucking talk about. I just have to sit there like an idiot. I don't know what's going to happen now. I don't know if I'll be able to afford to go to college at all. I'm stuck here, Rob. Stuck in Shitsville—*stuck*."

"Maybe you could get a scholarship?"

She laughed.

"Yeah—right. My grades are *horrible*. I barely go to class."

"What about a cheerleading scholarship?"

"I quit."

"Really?"

"Last week. I haven't told the girls yet."

"How come?" I asked.

"Because I need to make up a reason. I think I'll say that I hurt my ankle."

"No, I meant why'd you quit?"

"Don't laugh," she snapped.

"Who could *I* ever laugh at?"

She sat up and brushed the hair from her face.

"I quit because I don't have time to cheer anymore. I quit because I got a stupid fucking job at the Frostop on Route 60, because the stupid fucking lottery fired my dad for no reason and everyone is freaked we won't be able to pay our stupid fucking bills now."

Frostop—damn. I couldn't even imagine Ali *eating* at that place, let alone serving food to all those miners who stopped in between shifts.

"I *love* Frostop!" I said. "That's cool as hell."

Ali laughed as she leaned back into me.

"Whatever, if my friends knew they would fucking disown me. Why do you think I work all the way out in Barboursville?"

"They sound like pretty shitty friends."

She sighed. "Don't say anything. You're the only one who knows."

"I won't—I promise."

"Just *please* tell me if I start smelling like French fries, okay? I really don't want to smell like fucking French fries."

"I'll stay vigilant," I swore.

I could feel her body warming mine. The swing was still now, and we sat unmoving in the dark. I'd lost track of time. I'd lost track of everything.

"You know, I listened to the tape you made me," she said.

"*Really?* Did you like it? I wasn't sure about a few of the songs. You know, I only put that Ataris song on there because—"

"Rob," she said.

Her eyes met mine.

"Yeah?"

"Shut up."

She kissed me right then. She lit up my world.

FIVE

Parked Cars

1

Although Ali dropped off the cheerleading squad, she still swung enough weight at school to get a late transfer into my first-period class. This move was a big deal for me. I'd had plenty of girls try to get *away* from me, but Ali was the only one who ever tried to get closer.

Each morning in class, Ali passed me a note she'd scribbled on the cheesy pink paper she liked to use. These messages were little nothings—about what she was up to after school, a movie she wanted to see—but I carried them in my wallet like currency, rereading them incessantly through the rest of the school day.

The two of us had no other classes together. We were on separate schedules, and I was lucky if I even passed her in the hall. So while my teachers droned through boring lectures, I just read her notes. Then I read them again.

Although Ali and I spent the days apart, I couldn't seem to turn a corner without running into her friends. They were openly disgusted at the thought of us dating, and they couldn't help making shitty comments whenever I walked past.

But I didn't let it bother me. I mean, in a way I agreed with them—shit, I couldn't believe she was dating *me* either. But she was. And if Ali didn't care what her friends thought about it, why should I? As long as she could ignore them, I could too.

At first, the thought of Ali and me together seemed as off to my friends as it did to the cheerleading squad. She was above my pay grade, and I think they were nervous I was taking on more than I could handle.

But having a girl like Ali around came with benefits. For one thing, all guys know that attractiveness multiplies— pretty girls know pretty girls—so as long as Ali was dating a punk rocker, there was a chance that other chicks might decide to slum it with one of my friends.

Even more important than the possibility of girls was the reality of free fast food—Ali started showing up at band practice with carloads of Frostop milk shakes and fries. The seats of my van were littered with paper bags and wadded-up foil wrappers. The basement started smelling like a grease trap. It was amazing. As far as my gang was concerned, Ali ruled eternal.

She still partied with her friends every weekend, but Ali spent the rest of her free time with us. She went with us to bad movies and the crappy restaurants we loved. She took us seriously and always laughed at our dumb jokes. It wasn't long before she started ditching school on Tuesdays to go record shopping with the boys.

When we were alone, we only did two things: make out, or find places to make out.

It was too cold to skateboard in January, so the dudes

were usually at my house. With Ali's dad out of work, our options in the privacy department were limited. We generally retreated to the ancient sanctuary of the American teenager—the backseat.

We just kissed, mostly—I was afraid to try much more, scared I'd embarrass myself—I clawed and fumbled at her clothes, and my fingers inched nervously up her thighs. I was scared that she'd stop me. I was scared that she wouldn't.

On back-road turnoffs and empty church parking lots I lost myself. That Ford van was our hour-rate dive motel.

It became impossible to focus on anything else. If I wasn't around her, I *wanted* to be around her. I wanted to feel the way I did when she pulled me toward her—I needed it all the time, every minute. I wanted to watch the car windows steam up. I wanted I wanted I wanted.

I was completely obsessed.

This was an obsession that was different than music. I know I'm supposed to say music would always be my first love but shit, come on.

Of course I love music—*everyone* loves music! But music didn't wear tight black jeans. Music didn't have perfect 34-Ds I was allowed to feel up. Music touched me, but it never *touched* me—when Ali and I were alone, the music faded into the background.

Whether it was Bon Jovi, the Clash, or radio static, it didn't matter. Every moment with her sang.

*　　*　　*

Around the time we officially began dating, I started to have coughing fits whenever Ali lit up beside me. I could feel the smoke drift into my nose and down my lungs, causing these deep, sporadic coughs.

It was embarrassing as shit. She already knew that I wasn't cool enough to smoke—but being so uncool that I couldn't even handle *secondhand* smoke? How was that level of lameness even possible?

The cough began to follow me.

It stayed with me long after the butts of her cigarettes dimmed and died on the blacktop. Mom started asking if I felt okay. She said she heard me coughing in my bedroom some nights. She started to worry that I was getting sick.

I told her I was fine.

But the more I coughed, the harder it was to avoid her nagging about me being sick. I told Mom that it was probably allergies—*"No one has allergies in January"*—or that maybe spring was coming early.

Didn't that seem plausible? I mean, maybe it *was* allergies—there must be people in the world allergic to cigarette smoke. Incredibly unhip people, sure, but people nonetheless.

I finally told Ali that I'd diagnosed myself with a chronic cigarette smoke allergy. I said that she should quit smoking.

"Well, yeah, I could," she'd said, "but it would be easier if you just quit coughing instead. . . ."

We both had a pretty good laugh at that one.

2

The more I kept coughing, the less I was convinced it had anything to do with cigarette smoke. By February, I was at a point where I would break into these loud, room-clearing coughing fits; not just around smokers either. Now I coughed if I tried *any* physical act. It had nothing to do with exertion—I was just as likely to cough playing drums as I was simply walking up the stairs.

Mom kept nagging me to go to the doctor, and I kept brushing her off. The more I coughed, the more she nagged. It became a nightly debate at our house—Mom getting on my case, me saying that she was overreacting.

My dad finally told her that if I said I felt fine, then I felt fine. He gave me more credit than I deserved.

If I'd just listened to my body, maybe I would've known something was seriously wrong with me sooner than I did. It all seems so obvious to me now, but the truth is, if you woulda asked me back then, I would have told you there wasn't anything wrong at all.

In my experience, a cough or a sneeze was just a lead-in to a cold or flu or something. So I waited. And waited. But nothing came. Besides that cough, I felt fine. I felt *great*, actually; between the band and Ali, I was feeling no pain. I didn't have so much as a headache.

So it was easy for me to push the cough into the back of my mind. I didn't want to waste time going to some stupid doctor's appointment over a stupid cough. I had way more important shit to focus on.

So I didn't give it a second thought—at least until the blood.

* * *

On the morning I coughed up blood, I was sitting at the kitchen table, eating breakfast and listening to my mom bitch at me about going to the doctor. Dad was upstairs getting dressed, so I had no one to back me up.

Apparently, sometime in the night my cough got loud enough to wake up both my parents. In my mom's book, that settled it—I was going to the fucking doctor. But I still kept saying I felt *fine*. I didn't need to see a doctor.

"You've gotten the mistaken impression that I am *asking*," she said.

She ordered me to stay home from school and rest. She would call our family doctor once she got to work and schedule my appointment. He and his wife had been friends with my parents for years, so she didn't expect much of a wait.

I finally told her if I *had* to go to the doctor, fine—but I wasn't staying home. Not doing it. Nope. No way.

I hated school as much as any other kid—and *of course* I wanted to get rid of my cough—but it wasn't about school, and it wasn't about the cough. It was about Ali. If she was going to be at school, then so was I.

Mid-argument, I went into another coughing fit.

I dropped my spoon and leaned over the table as my body drove dry coughs through me with the force of an invisible fist on my back. I raised my hand to signal that I was fine, but then I kept right on coughing.

When I finished, I was sweating. I struggled to catch my breath. My eyes were fixed on the table.

"Yeah . . . yeah . . . okay . . ." I panted. "I'll . . . stay home. . . ."

Mom kept talking, but I was barely listening anymore.

My attention was on the empty cereal bowl in front of me, and the blood that was now inside it.

It wasn't a lot of blood—only about a teaspoon's worth, just little droplets that floated on my leftover milk like dark-red lily pads. Before Mom could see it, I took my spoon and swirled it in with the milk, diluting it all into a soft, safe pink.

As the blood disappeared, I tried to rationalize what had just happened.

This doesn't mean I'm sick, I thought. *In fact, this is proof that I'm not.*

I was sure that—because I wasn't sick—I had no phlegm or snot to cough up. So those dry, forceful coughs of nothing *must* have been *so* dry that this particular coughing fit irritated my throat, making me spit up a little blood. Because what else could it have been?

Only something I'd rather not think about.

Mom walked back upstairs. I could hear Nat watching MTV in the other room. I sat at the table, stirring. I looked out through the window at the new day ahead.

3

It looked like I was gonna be stuck at home for the rest of the week. Our family doctor had returned Mom's call but told her he was on sabbatical—I wasn't sure exactly what that meant, only that he wasn't at work. He promised that his receptionist would fit me in with the next available doctor. He said I needed to stay home until somebody checked me out.

I was balled up on the couch, watching *Ricki Lake* in

between coughs, when Ali stopped by. I hadn't talked to her much that week, so it was a surprise. A nice surprise.

We ended up driving by the park, in the small lot where the hiking paths ended. It was on the section opposite the playground and was almost always deserted. There were no other cars, no bikers, no joggers—nothing.

Ali put on our worn-out Bon Jovi mixtape, turned the volume low, and we climbed into her backseat.

We made out for hours, and I didn't cough at all. Ali had her shirt off, and her thighs rubbed against my love handles as we kissed. Bon Jovi was quiet now, and the sunlight beyond the windows had grown dim. I didn't notice.

She started unbuttoning my pants, and I started unbuttoning hers. I didn't know where it was going next, but it felt too awesome to stop.

She stopped.

"Oh shit," she whispered.

She jumped off me and started grabbing for her clothes.

"What is it?"

"*Cops,*" she hissed, strapping on her bra.

I jerked my head around—a black-and-white cruiser crept slowly into the entrance of the lot.

"Shit," I said, and started to cough.

"*Shit,* shut up! Shit!"

She climbed into the front seat. Her shirt was still unbuttoned, and her pants were halfway down her hips. I was still in the backseat with my head between my knees, coughing. I saw one of Ali's shoes lying on the floor.

She pulled out of the parking lot slowly, and the cops

followed us. We were driving through the neighborhood at about five miles an hour, with the cops stuck right on our bumper. I tried to get Ali to relax.

"It isn't like they saw us *doing* anything," I said. "How much shit can they give us for sitting in a parked car?"

"When the car has a ziplock full of pot in it, they can give us a *lot* of shit!" she said nervously.

"Jesus, how much pot do you smoke?"

"*Rob*, just hand me my shoe."

While she tried to slip the shoe on, she jerked the wheel—barely—and the cops hit their lights.

Their sirens squealed. Ali cursed and pulled over. I sat in the backseat, dumbstruck—I couldn't believe it. They'd pulled us over right in front of my fucking house.

The cops just sat in their cruiser. They turned off the siren, but the lights kept circling blue and red. Neighbors started to walk onto their porches. Soon, another police car arrived—"backup"—and the light show doubled.

Finally, an officer walked to the car.

Ali rolled down her window. She handed the cop her license. He didn't even look at it. He leaned down into the car, grinning.

"You swerved a bit back there, miss. You haven't been drinking today, have you?"

"No, sir."

"What about your little brother back there?" he said, nodding toward me.

"He doesn't drink."

"But you drink?"

"I . . . no, sir . . . I just meant he hasn't been drinking either."

He nodded. Then he told her to look into his eyes. He stared—hard.

"Your pupils look dilated," he said. "I'm gonna need you to step out of the car."

Ali did as she was told.

The other cops were out of their cruisers by now—watching my one-shoed, half-topless girlfriend do a field sobriety test in front of my entire block. Ali's shirt blew open in the wind as she touched her finger to her nose. I looked toward my front porch . . .

Fuck.

My parents were standing there, watching the entire scene unfold. If they hadn't already seen me sitting in the car, I know they saw me now—because Nat came out and stood beside them, laughing his ass off.

The cop led Ali back to her car.

I could hear the other cops laughing behind her. The doors of their cruisers slammed, and the lights died. Then they were gone.

Ali sat in the car with the engine still off. There was a rap at the window—*my* window. Dad and Nat stood on the curb, laughing. I sighed and rolled it down.

"Aren't ya gonna introduce me to this outlaw?" Dad said.

Mom had already walked back inside.

SIX

The Outline of a Heart

1

That first meeting between Ali and my parents could have been worse—the shit with the cops sucked, but we chalked it up to a misunderstanding (they'd thankfully missed the part where her shirt flew open). The air was getting unseasonably warm, and it seemed like winter had begun its long-overdue fade-out. Maybe the weather made everyone a bit more easygoing than usual.

Whatever the reason, all I know is that even though it was awkward at first, after a few visits my parents were as charmed by Ali as all of my punk friends had been.

My girlfriend and parents bonded over only one topic—my cough.

I thought it was stupid. What was the point of worrying about it? I was still coughing, wasn't I? Worrying didn't change shit.

But I did worry—secretly. Not about the cough, but about how it affected my drumming.

For a while, if I went into one of my fits we'd end practice. But that didn't last long—soon, instead of stopping practice, we'd just take little breaks until the coughing subsided. But shit, those breaks began to eat up half our rehearsal time!

So I finally decided I just needed to play through it.

I'd be coughing my lungs out, but I kept on playing. Eventually, the coughs would subside or the song would end—one way or the other, it would be fine.

*   *   *

I'd never really spent much time in the hospital. I'd had a few checkups, and I broke my arm once, but that's it. So when Mom and I went in for my first appointment on Monday, I felt a little uneasy.

But my anxiety may have had less to do with the cough than it did with my mom coming with me.

A mom driving her kid to the doctor doesn't seem like a big deal, but in those types of situations, *my* mom was a little intense. I knew she was worried about me, and I knew she wanted answers—and when she wanted them, she got them.

I also knew that the doctor would direct his attention to her, and not me. I'd just sit in the corner, embarrassed, and let the adults speak.

But whatever. The appointment was really for her, anyway. I figured that the cough would go away soon, doctor or no doctor. Mom was the one who was worried. So at least the appointment would get her off my back.

We walked into the lobby of the hospital, past the gift shop, toward the elevators. The place was full of old people—the staff, the doctors, the asses in those squeaky plastic waiting-room chairs—they were all so fucking *old*.

But none of them looked sick. Old as hell, sure—but not sick.

I don't mean sick like the way I was sick. I mean *sick* sick—with AIDS, or Ebola, or a gunshot wound. A few *sick* sick people had to be in there somewhere—it was a hospital, after all. The disinfectant smell made me think it was some sorta cover-up, like all the sickos were hidden away.

When we got on the elevator, I asked Mom what she thought. Where did she think they hid the goners, the real tragic cases?

"I *think* that my son shouldn't ask such horrible questions."

Mom checked me in with the receptionist herself. Our doctor's office had referred me to Dr. Sherman—she said that he would see us shortly.

Mom sat down right beside me, even though the waiting room was empty. We sat in silence for what seemed like an hour.

"Ali seems nice," she finally said.

"Yeah. She's rad."

"You two have big plans for Valentine's Day?"

"Come on, Mom—*Valentine's Day?* It's just an excuse for companies to sell chocolate and stupid cards."

"Well," she said, shrugging, "does *Ali* think it's stupid? Because I know I didn't when I was sixteen."

"I dunno," I mumbled.

"Maybe you should ask her what she wants to do— whether she thinks it's dumb or not. Women need to know they are heard. She'll appreciate it more than cards or chocolates, although chocolates are nice."

A fat nurse with a clipboard walked into the waiting room.

"*Robert Roofiz,*" she yelled.

Mom strutted past the nurse and through the door before I'd even made it out of my seat. *Women need to be heard,* I thought. *No shit.*

I sighed, stood up, and followed.

The nurse walked us into a bright white tile hallway. She had me kick off my shoes and step onto a scale—one hundred ninety-two pounds thin. I stood straight against the wall and she measured me—five feet six inches short. Then she led us into the exam room, flipping a red plastic flag outside the door to show it was occupied.

The exam room was so clean that it looked completely unused. A big exam table was in the corner, covered in a strip of parchment paper like the kind Mom used when she baked cookies.

The fat nurse sat me down. She took my temperature and my blood pressure, and then left the room. She told us that the doctor would be in shortly.

"You have to wait in a room just to wait in a room," I said.

"Welcome to real life, sweetheart."

An hour and a half later, there was still no doctor. I thought they'd forgotten about us. I wanted to leave. Mom refused. I lay down on the exam table and dozed to the buzz of the lights overhead.

I woke up when the heavy door slammed shut. I squinted into the fluorescent lights above me. I blinked until my eyes could focus on the blurry image of Dr. Sherman.

Dr. Sherman was about Mom's age, with little wire glasses and thinning brown hair. He had a mustard stain on his tie.

"So," he said, flipping through a chart, "I understand you've had a persistent cough?"

"Yeah," I said. "I cough, like, all the time. I don't spit anything up, no snot or nothing—just this cough."

He nodded. "Any other symptoms?"

"Not really," I said, and then Mom interrupted.

"*Actually*, he is having other symptoms—I would say that 'persistent cough' is the understatement of the year. These are *severe* coughing episodes; I mean coughs that wake everyone in the house up at night. He's in pain, even if he says he isn't. I can see him wince after each cough."

"Anything else?" Dr. Sherman said.

"He seems a little disoriented throughout the day and has been increasingly short of breath."

Disoriented—have I? I wondered.

"She's right, I have been really outta breath. I figured it was from the coughing."

Dr. Sherman told me to sit up straight. He looked into my eyes. He looked in my mouth. He made me say *aaaahhhh*. He ran his fingers under my jaw. He listened to my breath. He listened to my heart.

"Well," he finally said, "you don't seem to have strep, which is good."

"So what do you think is causing it?" Mom asked.

Dr. Sherman shrugged. "The cough may be a lingering symptom from a cold, or possibly allergies. Truthfully, I'm not too worried about it."

"But I *am* worried about it." She was speaking louder now. "He's been coughing for *weeks*—maybe longer. And I hear him wheezing when he walks up the stairs. He—"

"Robert is forty pounds overweight," he told her. "His weight, mixed with what I can only assume is a sedentary lifestyle, could be at fault for his shortness of breath. It may also have affected his ability to get over whatever brought his cough on in the first place."

He turned his attention to me.

"I'm going to write you a prescription for an antibiotic. Let's see if that helps knock out the rest of this cold." He paused. "I will also write a scrip for cough syrup . . . there is codeine in it. Do you know what codeine is?"

"No."

"*Sure* you don't. It should help with some of the pain you are feeling during these episodes. But *only* take it as directed—it is not a party favor, understand?"

"Uh, okay?" I said.

Dr. Sherman scribbled something onto his chart.

"If the cough hasn't cleared up by next week, you need to come back and see us—okay?"

Mom stood up behind him.

"Listen," she said, "he's *my* son. I've seen him with a cold, with strep throat—this is different."

"Well, your son apparently doesn't feel too sick to spike up his hair, so I don't think this cough is terminal just yet."

Before she could reply, Dr. Sherman grabbed her hand again, shook it, and left the room.

2

If I could tell myself I was okay, didn't that mean it was true?

I wasn't sure anymore. When I heard Mom raise her voice at Dr. Sherman, it wasn't anger that registered—it was concern. Fuck, man, it shook me up a little. The next day my life went back to its normal flow, but I found it harder to push the "symptoms" Mom spoke of out of my mind.

I went back to school while I waited for my antibiotics to kick in. Besides playing drums, and a few failed make-out sessions, I'd been completely inactive since my house arrest—so as I merged back into my old routine, I couldn't believe how much harder it was on me physically after only a week away.

I struggled to class in the mornings. My backpack felt heavier, as if someone had filled it with ball bearings. The hallways stretched out before me like some fun-house trick.

My breath was so thin that it shocked me. Simply making my way through the school took forever. This was just *walking* (more like strolling, even—I hadn't rushed even on my best days). Now I had to stop every few dozen feet and catch my breath. By the time I made it to my class-rooms, the hallways were completely empty. Even Ali, it seemed, gave up waiting for me against the first-period lockers. I stood outside the door until my breath got under control. Then I'd duck past the teacher and collapse at my desk.

I started to think that Mom was right about my attention span. I'd never really paid much attention in class, but now that I was back I found I couldn't concentrate even when I tried. I guess I hadn't noticed these changes when I was watching daytime television at home. But being at school meant learning—or at the very least, engaging, and I just couldn't seem to focus at all.

No matter how much I tried to pay attention, the information always became scrambled—twisting in my consciousness with random thoughts and images—a terrible pop song I'd heard, a day-old afterthought, a magazine cover, a car on the highway—every single thought and every single day blended and spun in my mind as one strange vision: a carousel dream that I could ride but never stop.

3

The cough syrup Dr. Sherman gave me came in a red bottle. The liquid inside of it looked thick and black—everything about it screamed *CAUTION*. I tried it a few times, just to see if it helped.

It tasted like turpentine; I could barely stomach two spoonfuls. It did ease the pain in my throat and chest a little, but it didn't stop the coughing. Mostly it made me feel fucked up, tired, and even more disoriented.

I wasn't sleeping much anymore.

In bed, all the thoughts of the day caught up with me. It was ironic, in a way. I spent my days exhausted, barely able to focus on the most simple tasks and conversations—but in the dark I couldn't shut my brain off.

Anxious thoughts came at me from every angle. I wished for sleep, struggled for it, but fighting just made things worse.

When the restlessness got to be too much, I'd lock myself in the small bathroom that was connected to my room. I sat on the cold tile floor and warmed myself with my small red hair dryer—the white noise was all that seemed to calm my head.

The sound magnified in the small space like I was in an echo chamber. I sat there for hours as the temperature rose in the darkness. I stared through the window and over my neighbor's rooftop, up toward the moon and where the stars should be. The mechanical hum of the dryer drowned the thoughts in my brain mercifully, rolling over each one like a calm, tideless ocean.

*   *   *

A week and a half later I went back to the doctor. Valentine's Day was only two days away. I took my mom's advice and asked Ali what she thought of it, to which she bitched about the horrible V Days of her past—so I knew I had to suck it up and take her out.

This time at the hospital, they stuck me with Dr. Dixon, a tall black guy with a heavy baritone voice. He listened more intently than Dr. Sherman had—to *me*, not just my mom—and didn't make any dick comments about my hair or weight.

But in the end, Dr. Dixon's opinion was the same as Sherman's—wait it out.

He told me to give it another week, keep taking the

cough syrup, and see if it subsided on its own. He said he'd give me a note for school, like that was the solution for the struggle of walking to class.

He said that if nothing changed in a week, he wanted to do a chest X-ray and look for signs of pneumonia, though he doubted that it was anything that serious.

4

Sappy card—check. Heart full of chocolates—check. Half-dozen (plastic) roses—check. Dinner reservations at the nicest restaurant in town—double check.

V Day was upon me, and I was armed with an arsenal of romantic crap.

Granted, the arsenal was supplied by *my mom* (lame!), who'd picked it all up at the pharmacy while waiting for my cough syrup to be refilled. I was embarrassed when she showed up with it all, but whatever. At least it was free.

Paul was putting on a special show that night, the Valentine's Day Massacre. He packed the bill with the most brutal bands he could find. Nat tried to get me to go with him, but I said I was too sick.

If the dudes knew that I was skipping a show to hang out with a chick—Valentine's Day or not—I would never hear the end of it. *What kind of pussy had I turned into?*

I called Ali at home.

"Hey," I said, "our dinner reservations are for eight thirty at Red Lobster. I figured I could pick you up a little earlier, and we could—"

"I was thinking we skip dinner."

"Why?"

"Because—my parents are out on a date."

"So?"

"*So,* they'll be gone all night."

"*Oh,*" I squeaked.

"So why don't you just come over? We can hang out here and stuff."

AND STUFF.

I cleared my throat.

"Right on," I said, as aloofly as I could. "That's fine, babe. Whatever you want."

"Okay, good. That's what I want."

She hung up the phone.

I was nerrrrrrvous nervous nervous, man.

Ali. Home alone. On Valentine's Day. I felt like the planets had aligned, and the chances of me finally getting laid were at their all-time high.

AND STUFF.

I checked my look in the mirror. I wanted to change my clothes, my hair, my face. I tore off my black T-shirt and put on a different black T-shirt. I paced around my bedroom. I paced around my bathroom. I paced until I was out of breath.

AND! STUFF!

I gathered up the candy and the plastic flowers. I grabbed the keys to the van. They jingled in my shaking hand.

Without thinking, I went into the kitchen and pulled my bottle of toxic cough syrup from the cabinet. I chugged eight good gulps, tensing my throat muscles so I wouldn't puke. I screwed the lid back on the bottle—I'd killed nearly half of it. I put it back in the cabinet and waited.

After about twenty minutes, I felt my nerves calm down. I felt better—tired, but better. *What was it that I was so nervous about?*

All of a sudden, I couldn't remember.

* * *

When Ali opened the door and saw me standing there with all that Valentine bullshit, she *screamed*—it was ridiculous.

She hugged me and kissed me and *pulled* me inside her house.

As she led me to the living room, there were no signs of her parents, brothers, or sisters anywhere. She took me over to the couch, where a rectangle-shaped gift was wrapped in her pink notebook paper. She'd written my name on it inside the outline of a heart.

I opened it slowly. It was a VHS tape—*Bon Jovi LIVE! Reading Festival, 1990.*

"I had to buy it," she said. "It was just so *us!*"

Goddamn it felt great to have an *us*.

We threw the tape in the VCR.

Jovi hadn't even gotten into their third song before we were fooling around. I was feeling about one swig of cough syrup away from passing out. But there is nothing—except maybe death—that cannot be overcome by teenage lust. So although my head felt foggy, Ali's body felt warm and perfect as it rubbed against me to those beautifully cheesy rock ballads.

When I tried to take off her shirt, she stopped me.

"You want to go in my bedroom?"

"Um—[*gulp*]—yeah . . . sure . . ." I said. I choked back a cough.

"You okay?"

I cleared my throat and promised I was fine. I would have promised anything at that point.

"I just don't want to get you sick," I told her. "I probably shouldn't even be kissing you."

Ali stood up and pulled me off the couch.

"Whatever you've got has got me too. Don't you know that by now?"

She led me into the bedroom.

Ali picked up a shirt off the floor and covered her table lamp. The light dimmed.

In the shadows she seemed older. She moved through her room with purpose. She led me to the bed and sat me down on its edge.

She shut the door. She locked it.

She stood in front of me and took off her shirt. I just sat there, staring up at her. She smiled at me and unhooked her bra.

I couldn't think or react. There were fireworks inside of my head. When she unbuttoned her jeans, I watched my left hand rise up and touch her hip. It was moving on its own.

I started coughing again. Ali stopped. I hacked until my face was burning bright red, and then sat there embarrassed, trying to catch my breath.

Ali eased me down on the bed.

"Take it easy. Just relax, okay? Don't worry about anything."

"Okay," I said.

When she started to undo my jeans I closed my eyes. I felt the weight of her body on mine, and the smoothness of her thighs around my waist as I sank down into the mattress.

I opened my eyes.

I counted the freckles above me, glowing and dimming and glowing again.

SEVEN

Kids Today

1

The day after Valentine's Day, I was *back* at the goddamn hospital.

Mom had been put in charge of a new project at the refinery, so it was a lot harder for her to get off in the middle of the day. This time I went alone.

They put me in the same exam room. The hospital had the same smell. The nurses were still overweight and detached.

Only the doctor was different. The receptionist told me which one I'd be seeing, but this time I didn't bother remembering his name.

I waited. I waited some more.

Finally, the doctor came in. I went over my whole spiel again— the cough, the symptoms, the progression, the other doctors—the whole exercise seemed so counterproductive. How did they not know this already? What the fuck was in my charts? Didn't these quacks even bother to read them?

After I rehashed my last two visits, I told him what had changed.

I was still coughing, and my other weird symptoms

seemed to be getting worse. My shortness of breath was worse than ever, and even the slightest activity had me pleading for air. I was confused a lot, and I'd been getting brutal headaches. I wasn't sleeping.

The doctor said that the lack of sleep might be causing my headaches.

"But what is causing this insomnia?"

"Probably the cough," the doctor said.

But he still couldn't tell me why I was coughing!

Unlike Dr. Dixon, this one didn't think the cough had anything to do with pneumonia. He saw no reason for me to get any X-rays.

He said that the symptoms were so strange, they could only be caused by a severe allergic reaction to *something*—maybe food, maybe linen or carpet, maybe some hidden mold, maybe an animal—he wasn't sure. Figuring out the culprit, he said, was up to me.

His best suggestion was to remove as many constants from my life as I could; family pets, bedsheets, clothes, carpet, all the food in the fridge. He said process of elimination was the best way to find out what was making me sick.

He told me to come back in two weeks.

That process of elimination started right away.

Dad ripped out my bedroom carpet using a box-cutter and a flathead screwdriver. Nat agreed to move into the basement temporarily and let me sleep in his bedroom. Mom went out and got new sheets for his bed, just to be safe.

These changes didn't produce any results. We couldn't find any mold, dander, or decay—we couldn't find anything suspicious at all. The symptoms continued.

A week passed.

I spent all seven nights awake, lying in my brother's bed coughing and confused.

What is going on with me? I wondered. *Am I going fucking crazy?*

2

A few days later the pain started.

It came out of nowhere—just like the cough, just like Ali, just like all of it. There was no lead-up, no sense to it. I simply woke up one morning—the same way I did every morning—and felt a pain in the bottom of my neck.

It wasn't pain like the cuts and bruises I got skating. It was a deep pain. It hurt all over my neck and shoulder, it hurt everywhere under my skin. It was inexplicable and constant—as if someone had slashed the nerve endings with a rusty ax while I was sleeping. This pain was all-encompassing.

I'd never felt anything like it. It was completely fucking brutal. I still had three days until my follow-up appointment—my parents told me to stay home.

That was fine. I didn't want to be at school anymore. I didn't want to move. The clouds in my mind had turned black again. I couldn't think, I couldn't reason—something inside of me had finally broken.

No one knew what to do. I looked fine; there were no bruises or injuries. I wasn't sore to the touch. The pain was invisible.

Alone in my house, I started taking Advil by the handful. Taking and taking and taking those pills, sucking on the coating like it was candy. I drank the cough syrup freely now, eager for the codeine to make me numb.

None of it helped much, but I didn't know what else to do. I'd lie in bed all day, trying to figure out what the hell I coulda done to hurt myself this bad—I couldn't remember. The constant quality of the pain was making me feel crazy. My memory was as unclear as everything else. I couldn't remember the past, and I didn't have the energy to think of tomorrow.

All I could focus on was *now*, where I was living inside the pain.

I wanted to be alone. The pain and the cough, the sleepless nights—it was all too much. Anytime I talked to anyone—on the phone or in person—my fuse was nonexistent. I was miserable and made sure everyone knew it.

So I just stayed in bed, rolling over, whining (and finally—crying) while red sirens screamed their endless *wampwampwamp* in my brain.

Days, nights, and mornings—the pain was always with me. It pushed me past sleeplessness and into full-blown insomnia. In the lifeless house of night, pain distorted my every thought.

It was a lonely place to be.

There were no dreams and no nightmares. I would have welcomed nightmares, if they meant sleep. But all that came was time—endless hours of dark.

Some nights, I convinced myself that I was imagining everything—people did that, right? Convinced themselves that they were sick to the point their own bodies believed it? I started seriously considering the possibility that I was losing my mind.

Fear, paranoia, and resentment were part of my every thought. It was like a strange acid in my neck was seeping into my brain—it was the acid that kept me awake.

The entire world seemed asleep. My parents and my brother, my gang, my teachers, Ali and her shitty friends, Johnny Ramone, Britney Spears, George Bush—millions and trillions of assholes everywhere—and they could all sleep.

Everyone slept but me. I hated them for it—silently— as I lay there alone with my thoughts and my pain.

It was horrible company to keep.

3

I'd given up on doctors.

Fuck them—fucking quacks. *Three months* to get rid of a cough? That seemed like some pretty shitty medical care, even in West Virginia. If it wasn't for the pain, I don't think I would have bothered going to my next appointment. But it forced me—*forget about the cough. Forget all of it. Just do something about this pain.*

Nat offered to drive me to the hospital. I'd been so laid up, I don't think he believed I could make it across town. But I said no—I was too miserable to accept any help.

I felt like they were just patronizing me—I was sure that no one really believed there was anything wrong with me. I'd convinced myself that they all thought I was a fake.

*   *   *

My faith in the hospital was nonexistent. Like I said, at this point I didn't even pay attention to names of doctors or medications, I just went through the motions. *When someone makes me feel better,* I said to myself, *I'll waste time remembering names.*

But then, there was Doctor . . .

Actually, screw him. I remember his name, but I won't say it. He doesn't deserve to have his name in a book, even one like mine. He doesn't deserve a legacy, even if it's that of a righteous prick.

So I'll refer to him by a pseudonym, one that I find much more fitting: Dr. Adolf Fuckface.

Dr. Adolf Fuckface—forever an asshole. Thin, graying hair combed down on his smug rat face. Thin lips frozen in an eternally smug grin.

Dr. Fuckface. Probably a child molester and a wife beater, probably a Nazi sympathizer and a Scientologist. He is definitely a fucking Republican. I bet he even loves Clapton's solo stuff.

Do you remember me, you worthless quack?

I seriously doubt it.

Because I vividly recall how he looked at me as soon as he entered that exam room. I was hunched over on the table, with my bleached spikes facing the door—a sweaty, pale boy in big smudged glasses, wearing a Black Flag T-shirt and ripped jeans.

Dr. Fuckface looked up from his clipboard as I croaked a hello. He regarded me with the kind of look you might give a public restroom—disgusted, irritated, and then dismissive.

I began at the beginning.

I started reliving my symptoms, going all the way back before the cough. He didn't ask any questions or make any notes; he didn't refer to my chart at all. He just leaned against the wall and looked at me. He had dismissed me the second he saw me.

But if he thought I was some loser freak—so what? I still needed help.

So I kept going. For once I was speaking candidly about the pain, the insomnia, and how hard it was for me to breathe. I asked him if he could do that chest X-ray. I asked him to do any tests he could—*do all the tests! Do everything!*

I was desperate. *Can't you see the pain I am in?* I wondered, rubbing my neck and shoulder. *Can't you help me?*

When I had finished, Dr. Fuckface just stood there, rubbing his chin.

"What is this *look* you're going for here, Robert?"

"What?"

"That T-shirt you have on. That *hair*—I mean, why would you do that to your hair? How *old* are you? My God, kids today look like circus clowns."

I wasn't sure what to say.

"Uh, okay? Not sure what my shirt has to do with the pain in my neck. I've been coming here for so long, and nothing has helped. They were supposed to do X-rays, and haven't, and I'm *still* sick."

He waved his hand insistently. "You don't *need* an X-ray. If you did, don't you think we would have done one by now? What you *need* to do is take the medication your previous doctor prescribed. Then come see us again if—"

"I DID TAKE THE MEDICINE! I took *all* the medicine; I tried everything they told me to try! *Nothing* helped! *Please* do the X-rays. Change my medication. Do *something*. I can't sleep. I can barely breathe."

I was panting now, and the air in the room seemed thick. Then, softly, I told him something I hadn't told anyone.

"I'm scared, man. I'm *freaking out*—please do something."

He cleared his throat.

"As I was saying before your tantrum, if you take the previously prescribed medication—*as directed*—I am confident the cough will subside."

"What about the pain?" I pleaded. "This weird pain in my neck—*nothing* makes it go away! It isn't normal."

Dr. Fuckface shook his head. "May I be frank, Robert?"

I was done. I just looked at the floor. I was done.

"I think what you need to do is start acting like a man. No medication or X-ray is going to help with that. I mean, listen, *I* have pain too—right here, in my knee, an old tennis injury—but do you know what I do? Do you know what *you* need to do? *DEAL WITH IT.* You are behaving like a little girl. You need to *deal with it*, Robert."

I sat there shaking. I hung my head when he left the room. I never saw him again. I never got a chance to tell him just how wrong he was. I just sat there, feeling like a complete nothing.

* * *

I wasn't thinking, I was just driving. I was scared—once I'd said it out loud, I couldn't deny it anymore.

I was fucking scared.

It wasn't until I passed the cemetery that I realized I was driving toward Ali's house. The two of us had barely talked lately, because I'd been so miserable to be around. Our last conversation had ended with her hanging up on me. Whenever I spoke, the poison inside of me seemed to come out.

I really had the feeling I was going down, man. I knew I should turn my car around. Only a coward would pull a poor girl onto a sinking ship. Only the most selfish prick would even consider it—but in the end, I just couldn't help myself.

I stood outside of her house. I banged on the door, yelling her name to the window above like an imitation Marlon Brando.

Ali finally answered the door. I saw her eyes widen.

"Shit, Rob, are you okay?"

"Why does everyone keep asking me that?"

She didn't answer me.

"I'm fine, I guess. I don't know anymore," I mumbled. I didn't realize that I was crying.

Ali wrapped her arm around my back and slowly walked me inside.

Our hearts beat beside each other on top of her unmade bed. She lay behind me, one arm around my chest and one on my neck as I spoke. It all poured out, between sobs and coughs—I told her about the pain and sleepless nights. I told her that I was scared I might be going crazy. I told her I was losing my grip.

I went on and on, until there were no words left. I had no more excuses, apologies, or concessions left to give. I was empty now.

Ali rubbed my neck. Her breasts pressed against my back, rocking in and out with her breath. Her body pushed against mine—leading it—until my shallow breaths flowed in tune with her own.

She told me it was okay. That everything was going to be okay.

And for the first time in a long time, I slept.

EIGHT

The Days Just Get Away from You

1

A few days after my visit with Dr. Fuckface, the pain stopped. It simply disappeared, as mysteriously as it had arrived.

My other symptoms lingered, but the pain—that *horrible* pain—was gone. I started leaving the house again. I started feeling like *myself* again.

None of it made sense.

Had I imagined it? Was it just growing pains? Lovesickness?

Ridiculous theories like this were discussed openly in my house, each resulting in a similar answer—if I was feeling better, then who cares?

On my second day back at school, we got home to find Brody standing on our porch. He was pacing manically, clutching his messenger bag. He told us that he had news—big news. He couldn't keep still.

We didn't have a band practice scheduled, but we still went down to the basement to talk about whatever had him so excited. Pillows and a comforter covered the love seat where Nat had been sleeping. Headphones were plugged into the stereo—I realized that I couldn't remember the last time I'd listened to music.

Nat and I watched Brody open his bag.

He pulled out a large white envelope, and then a smaller one. Both had been opened. He pulled a piece of paper out of the small envelope, flattening it on the floor.

"*Read,*" he said excitedly.

Nat and I looked down.

Brody,

I was pleased to receive your music and letter, thank you for the kind words. I thoroughly enjoyed the tape, as did my staff. To my knowledge, we've never had a band from West Virginia on the tour before. It seems there is a first time for everything.

See you this summer,

Kevin Lyman

Warped Tour

His name was signed at the bottom. Nat picked up the letter and read it again. I was speechless. Brody opened the large envelope before either of us could respond.

THE AGENCY GROUP was in big, bold print on the top of each page. It looked like some sort of form. There were spaces for names and Social Security numbers.

"Is this a contract?" asked Nat.

"It's an *offer*. Keep reading."

When we got to the last page, it made sense:

The Agency Group (TAG) submits to offer "Defiance of Authority (DOA)" two hundred dollars ($200) for live performance at the following Warped Tour appearances:

July 11: GTE Virginia Beach Amphitheater,
   Virginia Beach, VA
July 12: US Phoenix Center, Bristow, VA
July 13: US Tweeter Center, Camden, NJ
July 14: IC Light Amphitheater, Pittsburgh, PA
July 15: OFF
July 16: Asbury Park Lot, Asbury Park, NJ
July 17: Tower City Amphitheater, Cleveland, OH

I saw the offer shaking in my brother's hand. He looked up at Brody.

"We did it?" he asked tentatively.

"We did it!" Brody yelled.

Nat started laughing.

"We did it! We fucking did it!"

"We are going on tour!"

"THE WARPED TOUR, dude! Fuck!"

"It's *so* on!"

"Fuck! It is *so* fucking *on*!"

We were going on tour we were going on tour we were *going on tour*!

None of us could believe it. We'd never even played out of state before. We didn't have a record deal, or even a record. But now, we were invited to be part of the crown jewel of punk rock concerts, the *biggest festival tour in the world*!

We did it. It worked. We fucking did it.

At the time, I couldn't fully appreciate how insane it was that our little band got an offer like that—it was like we hit a grand slam on our first time at bat. But back then, it seemed a lot less like luck, and a lot more like destiny.

2

Word about our big break spread through the local punk scene quickly—mainly because we told anyone who would listen.

We were the first band from West Virginia to ever get invited on the tour—I couldn't remember ever feeling so proud. We started getting asked to play more shows—not just in West Virginia, but in other states too. Nat was looking at maps, talking about the possibility of booking more gigs around Warped Tour. Maybe we'd just tour all summer! Maybe we would tour *forever*!

We all had the urge to go out and play. Even me. Even as bad as I felt. I was now technically a professional musician—and as a professional, I felt like I needed to get off my ass and go play a show.

We were asked to play with an up-and-coming emo band at the VFW Hall in Charleston. The show was the following Friday, and super-late notice, but Ashley said the band was getting huge—which meant a crowd of new faces for us to rock off. It was as good a time as any to jump back into things. I felt a nagging sense that there was no time to waste.

It was our first out-of-town gig.

We loaded up the tour van with our instruments like always, and filled the leftover space with freeloaders from the local scene—Ashley, Paul, Tyson, Brody, Jamie, and Angela crammed into the seats. I'd invited Ali to come, but she said she couldn't. She was busy with her friends or something.

Charleston is about an hour east of Huntington. But on that night it seemed farther—beyond the lights of town, the world outside of our crowded van seemed strange and new. Everyone was excited. We blasted a Face to Face CD loud enough that everyone could sing along without feeling embarrassed.

The Charleston VFW was a crappy, one-story building on the far side of the capitol. The show promoter met us in the parking lot. He shook everyone's hand and really kissed my brother's ass. He offered to help us with our gear. The parking lot was full of kids, hanging out before the bands started.

It was different, but the same.

The only thing that *definitely* wasn't the same was the chicks—they had real live punk rock girls here. They sat on the hoods of cars drinking, laughing in the shadows on the walls. As I carried my snare drum inside, I had a vision of the vampire girl who'd sold me my records a lifetime ago. Would she have ever guessed she'd met a future punk rock star?

As I walked out for the next load, I made eye contact with a group of girls. I tried smiling, but it was no use— the headlining band had shown up. All females were suddenly occupied.

Since Paul wasn't promoting, he found himself with little to do. The two of us stood outside, waiting for our set time, staring at the golden rooftop of the capitol.

"Where's Ali?" he asked.

"With her friends, I guess. She's been hanging with them a lot lately. I think she's getting sick of me being sick."

"Shit, she'd better shape up before your tour starts. Don't she know that they make girls like her in Pittsburgh and in New York and in Jersey? Plenty of them will be happy to hang out with y'all this summer, I guarantee it."

We laughed.

"You're gonna come with us, right?" I asked.

Paul stared at the capitol, squinting in an expression between longing and disgust. He just shrugged.

"Come on, man. You are. You know we need you around."

"I'll go, I'll go. Just don't drop dead first."

*   *   *

We played the setlist from our last YWCA gig. Now it seemed so different—the room was packed with strangers, dancing and pushing each other along with our music. It wasn't like a hometown show—these people didn't know us, but they were still *feeling* us—they were into our shit.

I hit the drums weakly, struggling for breath—but it didn't matter. My throat hurt from coughing, but I didn't care. The crowd gave me their energy, and I gave it right back—we were all gears in one badass rock 'n' roll machine. It was an *incredible* show, one of the best I'd ever played.

Until we got to our fifth song. That's when I puked all over myself.

I don't know what happened, exactly. I was gasping for breath, struggling through the second verse, and then all of a sudden, I started vomiting. I hadn't been feeling nauseous, or anything. I was confused, but all I could think to do was finish the song.

So I turned my head to the side and barfed all over my pants and high hat—but I kept on playing.

After the song ended, I felt super dizzy. Little flashbulbs popped in my vision. Paul rushed onto the stage with water. He rubbed my back and started to ask me if I was okay, but as we looked down at this pile of dark red puke, we both registered that I most definitely was not okay.

Nat walked back to the drums. He was talking to me, but I couldn't tell what he was saying. I leaned over my snare drum, dazed and still trying to catch my breath. The look on his face scared me.

He went to the microphone and said something else. Before I knew it, he'd removed his guitar and he and Paul were walking me through the crowd, into the night and toward the van.

Nat opened the door and I climbed in the back. I collapsed onto the bench seat. Nat was talking, but I still couldn't concentrate well enough to make much out. Behind him, I heard yelling.

Brody had walked out behind us. His bass was still strapped to his neck. He and Paul stood in the parking lot arguing—Brody was pissed that we'd ended the show early.

My hearing began to fade back in, and I made out the words "small time" and "bullshit" in Brody's high-pitched voice—before Paul pushed him. Brody stormed back inside.

More people emptied into the lot. The promoter came outside and walked toward the van. Nat stood in front of the door.

"Look," he told the promoter, "I know we ended early—but my bro is fucking sick. We're done. If anyone's pissed, tell them to talk to me."

"*Whoa*, easy, easy . . . *pissed? Who's pissed? That was great!*"

Nat looked back at me, confused. The promoter walked to the open door and picked up my limp hand from the seat. He shook it up and down.

"However you did that, man—it was fucking *brilliant!*"

"Huh?" I moaned.

The promoter laughed.

"*Come on,*" he said. "Puking and playing! Playing and puking! *Fuck!* That was the most punk rock thing I've ever seen in my life."

3

I asked Nat not to say anything about the show once we got home. At this point, what difference would it make? After a day or so I started feeling a lot better. No nausea, no nothing. At least, not until we went out for a family dinner at the nicest restaurant in town, the one I'd tried to pamper Ali at on Valentine's Day—Red Lobster.

It was a send-off dinner for Mom—she'd got put on another new work project, and this one would take her to the company's other refinery in Findlay, Ohio. It was slated to take up to a month to complete. She was leaving town the next day.

We told our parents about the tour offer. They seemed skeptical, but they didn't dissuade us from going. I don't think they ever got tired of seeing us excited about life.

It was a nice night, and a nice time together, but on the drive home, it happened again.

Out of nowhere, I started spewing eleven-dollar shrimp all over the fucking backseat. Mom screamed. Dad almost wrecked the car.

When I was done puking, I put my head in my sweaty hands. I didn't want to face anyone. I stayed that way until we were home.

It was the second pair of shoes I had to wash that week.

*   *   *

I had pain again.

It was different this time—a stabbing pain in my left hip, right below my belly. It made me limp a little, but I was walking pretty slowly those days, anyway. So I tried not to make much of a fuss about it. It wasn't as severe as the pain in my neck, at least.

When Mom called me into her bedroom, I thought she was going to ask me about my limp. She didn't. Her suitcase was packed on the bed. Dad sat in front of the TV in a T-shirt and underwear, polishing his shoes.

Mom stroked her hand down the side of my hard yellow hair. She tried to meet my eyes, but I looked away, embarrassed.

"I feel horrible for leaving you this way, I'm a horrible mother."

"*Jesus Christ*, Mom."

"Do you remember my doctor—Stephanie Hallbeck?" she asked. "You met her last year, at the Christmas party."

I shrugged.

"Well, I just got off the phone with her. I explained the situation and she fit you in for an appointment, next Tuesday. Your father has agreed to take you."

"Mom, I don't want to go to any more doctors—there's literally no point."

"Tell that to the guys who are gonna have to detail my vomit-filled car tomorrow," Dad said.

"Whatever, y'all don't understand. Those doctors don't even *listen* to me."

"Stephanie is *my* doctor—I trust her. Just please let her look you over. She can at least do the tests that the other doctors mentioned."

"Maybe she'll throw in a free Pap smear," Dad said.

Mom threw a roll of pantyhose from her suitcase at him. She missed.

She would be gone before I woke. She asked me to hug her. I rolled my eyes, but I did. She kissed my forehead and said she would be back soon. She told me not to exert myself the way that I had been lately. When she told me she loved me, I felt too embarrassed to say it back.

4

The day of my appointment was a good day. I'll always be thankful for that.

Normally I wouldn't have remembered it. That's how it goes—the days just get away from you, burning like matches in a matchbook, blazing alone and then as one single flame. Melding together until they just burn out.

So I feel lucky to carry that day. I feel lucky to remember.

I didn't need to go to school. I was working on an essay for English about punk rock, but otherwise, my only reason for going was to see Ali. But I wanted to see her. I always wanted to see her.

So I got up, showered, and tried my best to look cool. I wore a pair of black jeans and my high tops, a white AFI shirt and the thin gray Vans jacket I knew she dug. When Nat saw me come down the stairs with my backpack, he just shook his head.

"Goin' today?"

I nodded.

"Well, fuck it. Come on."

He grabbed his keys.

Spring was finally here. The sunrise lit our horizon like a blue-pink cotton-candy sky. Nat and I rolled down our windows, and the morning smelled like fresh-cut grass. Our neighborhood was shot through with living color.

Nat walked beside me through the school parking lot and into the front hall. I limped in short, slow strides. My left leg dragged a little. He slowed his pace. Paul offered to carry my backpack, but I told him that I was fine. I had to stop twice before we made it inside.

Ali smiled when she saw me. She looked perfect in her tight green (low-cut) sweater and black choker necklace. She was glad that I was going back to the doctor—I told her it was just going to be a quick checkup.

"Maybe we can do something afterward?" I asked.

"I have to work tonight."

"Okay."

"Can you come see me at work? On my smoke break?"

"Fuck *yes*, I can," I said, smiling now.

A nerdy Filipino kid named David sat beside Ali. He had second-period photography with Paul and was always fiddling with a camera on his desk. That morning, he asked Ali for permission to take our picture.

"For what?"

"Just a class assignment," he said. "We're learning how to develop black-and-white."

She looked over at me. "Sure, why not."

I moved to where David had been sitting and scooted the chair right beside her.

"Guess I'll finally be able to prove I got a cheerleader to dig me once," I joked.

She put her arm around my left shoulder.

"They'll believe you, drummer boy. Trust me."

We looked toward the camera, laughing together, and held our hands up in mock heavy-metal rock horns.

That moment is frozen flat, one-dimensional.

The color of the morning has faded. The day exists only in black-and-white. Me, on that last day with a beautiful girl at my side, smiling her smile for me one last time.

NINE

Dead Boys

1

Dad had never taken me to the doctor before. Not once. To him, checkups fell under the same category as guidance counselors, shopping, and church—i.e., *Shit Your Mother Deals With*—so our ride to the hospital felt a bit strange for us both.

Dr. Hallbeck's office was in a part of the hospital that I'd never been to before. The move felt like progress. Her waiting room was filled with women wearing suspicious looks.

When the nurse called my turn, Dad looked over at me.

"Coming?" I asked.

"I guess your mother would kick my ass if I didn't, huh?"

"Definitely, dude."

He put down his magazine and followed me back.

I recognized Dr. Hallbeck once I saw her. Middle-aged, graying hair but still pretty-ish, if not for her glasses (they were even bigger than mine). She was the first doctor who showed any genuine concern—and not just for me. She was alarmed that other doctors in her hospital had been so flippant with my treatment.

"Your lungs sound horrible," she said, with her stethoscope pressed against me. "I am going to order that chest X-ray right now. If this is pneumonia, it is a severe case. If the X-ray shows what I think it will, we need to start treating it right away."

When we left the exam room, Dad and I both shook her hand.

"Finally, we're getting somewhere," Dad said.

"Yeah, and it only took them *four months*."

He patted my back and chuckled. We went looking for the X-ray lab.

* * *

X-ray was located in the basement of the hospital, with all the other radioactive machines. There were no magazines to read, just a waiting room made of the hard plastic chairs you'd expect to find at the DMV. Everything about it was utilitarian. It was clear that unless patients *needed* to be on this floor, they weren't.

Another nurse called me back. This time I asked Dad to wait.

The radiology lab was dark, and messier than I would have expected.

There was a long white table in the middle of the room, and a whiteboard in the corner. The tech told me to remove my shirt and glasses and stand against the board. I felt embarrassed to be shirtless in front of her. My chest and shoulders drooped like a melting vanilla ice cream cone. She told me to straighten my back, then to clasp my hands and raise them over my head.

I could hear the X-ray machine power up. A light shone on my pale stomach. I thought I might feel something, but I didn't.

"Breathe in," the tech said. "Good. Now hold your breath, hollldddddd . . ."

The machine made a soft sound. She told me I could drop my hands and gave me a minute to catch my breath. Then she told me to turn to my right side and repeat. Then the left side—and that was it. I was done.

"That was fast," Dad said when I returned to the waiting room. "How'd it go?"

"Fine, I guess. They told me to come out here and wait."

"Well, big boy—let's wait."

*   *   *

We sat there for hours.

Other patients came down periodically, sitting near us until they were called back for this scan or that one. We never saw them afterward. I wondered if they'd forgotten about us. I wondered if we should just leave.

I stood up and headed down the hall to try to figure out what the holdup was. The entire floor seemed deserted. I held on to the wall and panted down to the corner of the hallway.

I saw an old man outside one of the rooms. He was lying flat in a hospital bed, covered in a thin white sheet.

He wasn't moving. A nurse must have sat him there, the way you would an empty grocery cart. Behind the double doors, machines growled.

I left the man and walked slowly back.

"Any luck?" Dad asked. I sat down beside him and wheezed.

"Nope . . . you . . . ?"

"A few nurses walked by. I stopped them, but they wouldn't talk. All they said was we need to keep waiting."

"But we've been here *all day*."

"I know, I know," he said, leaning back into his chair. He'd removed his blazer, and the collar around his neck was now open.

Thirty minutes later, two nurses walked past us. Dad waved them down. Hesitantly, they stopped. He approached them. When he spoke, they didn't meet his eyes.

"The name is Rufus. We had an X-ray done *hours* ago. I just wanted to see if we can get out of here, or . . ."

I noticed one of the nurses, the younger one, staring at me.

Our eyes met—then all of a sudden, her lip trembled. She looked like she was crying. She took off down the hall. Dad looked at the other nurse.

"We are truly sorry for the wait," she said flatly, ignoring the other nurse's outburst. "The doctor will be with you in just a moment. Please *do not leave* until you have seen the doctor."

"Sure. Thanks," Dad mumbled, the color draining from his face.

He walked back over and sat down.

"*Weird*, man," I said.

He didn't answer me.

He just stared at the door of the X-ray lab.

A few moments later, the same nurse motioned us toward the lab.

We followed her into the X-ray lab, and then through a side door into a room with control panels and computer monitors. Then she ushered us into a room beyond the room.

It was clear that this room was not intended to receive guests. It was cluttered with papers, X-ray film, and coffee cups. A large desk ran along the far wall—a man sat behind it. The stacks of paper on the desk nearly hid him from view. He pushed a few folders out of his way.

He introduced himself as Dr. Houston, the hospital's chief radiologist. We sat across from him, anxious. Why were we back here? I waited for some kind of news. My leg was twitching.

"We reviewed your X-rays. Now, initially we were looking for signs of pneumonia. What we found was . . . different."

Dr. Houston clicked a button, and the far wall lit up like a bug zapper.

X-rays of what must have been my body were stuck to the lit-up wall. I looked inside myself—I saw a dark shadow in the middle of my body.

Dr. Houston was still talking. "What we seemed to have found is some sort of mass in the middle of the chest cavity. This explains the shortness of breath, and the coughing as well."

"Mass?" I said. "What does that even mean?"

Dr. Houston massaged his temples.

"Well, we won't know until we've done more tests. But from what I see here, and considering your age and speaking freely, my initial reaction would be that it may be a form of lymphoma."

Dad moved to the edge of his chair.

"Speak fucking English," he snapped.

Dr. Houston cleared his throat.

"I shouldn't make any assumptions until we run more tests."

"Lymphoma?" I said. "Is that, like, leukemia?"

"Sort of. The two diseases are often paired."

"Wait," Dad interrupted. "Are you saying this is cancer?"

Dr. Houston didn't answer. He just sighed and stared at his desk, as if he were searching for words in all that clutter.

Cancer?

"Is this—*mass*—inside of me like a tumor or something?"

The doctor rubbed his eyes with the sleeve of his jacket. Then he looked me square in the eye.

"We don't know, Robert. But we will find out—fast. You are very lucky you got this X-ray. Your lungs look on the verge of collapsing."

"Does my son have cancer?" Dad said. His voice was on edge.

I'd never heard him sound that way. Nervous. *Scared.*

"Mr. Rufus . . ." *Sigh. Pause.* "I am sorry. Yes, lymphoma is a type of cancer that is common in children and young adults. As you see from the X-rays this mass is localized to . . ."

His words drifted farther away from me.

They continued to talk, Dr. Houston pointing at X-rays. I felt weightless—I was sinking in on myself. I felt blank. I thought of all those machines outside, the white noise of their engines—blank and empty—calling to me. I sat there expressionless. I slipped into the hum.

2

They didn't want me to leave the hospital, but there was no real reason for me to stay—it was almost eight now, and most of the staff was already gone. So they finally told us to meet back at Dr. Hallbeck's office first thing in the morning, so she could take us to Oncology.

I didn't care, either way. I existed on a calm plain of shock. I had the night to "get things in order," as if that was an obvious process.

On the drive home, neither of us knew what to say.

"You hungry?" Dad finally asked.

"Sure."

"What'll it be, big boy? Anything you want."

What I wanted didn't seem to be something that came in a takeout container so I said pizza would be okay.

We got to the house around nine. The delivery guy from Gino's was standing like a clown in his yellow-red uniform. He held a stack of pizza boxes that reached over his head. Dad looked at the food like he'd forgotten he ordered it.

"Right. Hold on a second, buddy." He pulled out all the cash in his wallet and handed it to the delivery guy.

"For real?" the pizza guy asked. Dad nodded.

"Just help me carry this shit inside."

We had seven pizzas, three packs of garlic bread, and two two-liters—but neither of us knew what we should say to Nat. He stood before the stack of boxes, confused.

Dad tried to explain what the doctor had said, leaving out the words *tumor* and *cancer*. Dad called it "a thing with my lymph nodes," and told him that I was going back in the morning.

I couldn't listen anymore. My hands were getting shaky.

I threw five slices onto my plate and went down to the basement. I didn't know where else to go.

I sat down there alone, eating pizza on the stairs, trying to get my thoughts together. Through the door, I could still hear Dad and Nat talking. I didn't know anything about cancer—except that lots of people died from it. I knew that it was *BAD*.

People with cancer get chemo, lose their hair, puke—I had the base-level knowledge that any American TV viewer has, but that was it.

I didn't know what cancer really *meant*.

It was like some secret disease; people talk about cancer treatment, but they don't talk about the cancer. *Does the cancer hurt? Will I feel it inside of me? How does it kill?*

The basement door opened. My brother slowly came down the stairs.

"Hey," he said, sitting down beside me.

"Hey."

"Well, *this* is fucked up."

"Yeah. I know."

"You think they'll make you get chemo, or something?"

I shook my head. No one knew anything yet. Nat stood up and began pacing around the room, drumming on his thighs.

"Well, look, even if you *do* have to get chemo—fuck it. You know? I mean, you can't be *that* sick—we just played a fucking show, man!"

"Yeah. I guess so."

"*See!* So even if you get chemo, I bet it won't be that big of a deal. Ya know? Shit, you'll get to miss a ton of school and maybe you'll even lose weight. By the time Warped Tour rolls around, your hair will be grown back and you'll be fucking *fine*."

The TOUR—I hadn't even thought about that.

"Maybe. I hope so."

I stood up from the stairs. Nat walked closer to me.

"You're going to be fucking *fine*, dude. This is *all* going to be *fucking fine*."

I nodded. "Yeah. Okay. It'll be fine."

"Fuck it."

"Fuck it."

The basement door opened again. Dad stood at the top of the stairs, looking down at the two of us.

"Your mother is on the phone," he said, "she asked if she could talk to you."

I walked up the stairs and took the receiver. I was breathing heavily. Mom wasn't crying, which was good. If she had been crying, I think I would have finally lost it.

She said that she was coming home.

* * *

125

It was ten thirty. Ali was still at work. I knew I had to tell her, or at least tell her *something*.

I looked up the number for the Route 60 Frostop in the yellow pages. Some flunky answered, and I told him to put Ali on. I told him it was an emergency.

She took the receiver out into the parking lot. I imagined her there, in the glow of the streetlights, staring at the empty space where I should have been parked.

I surprised myself by saying it out loud—*they think I have cancer.*

Ali screamed and screamed. I tried to calm her down, I told her it would all be fine. I told her the same things Nat told me—but she kept crying, apologizing for nothing in slurred tones. I felt the tremor in her voice when she spoke.

Eventually, she ran out of tears. She grew silent. We just sat there on the line, me in my bedroom, and her in that lonely parking lot, stained with puddles of tears for me.

"I love you I love you I love you I love you," she swore.

"I know," I said, "I know. Everything is cool—I promise. Calm down. I'll call you after my appointment tomorrow. It might not be a big deal—okay? The appointment is way early, so I'll probably just see you back at school."

"Okay. It might not be a big deal. I'll see you at school."

I don't know if either of us really believed it.

3

I heard Mom's car pull in around three in the morning. I'd spent the last few hours on AOL, e-mailing Paul and the few other friends that I had. I told them as little as possible. After Ali, I just couldn't make another phone call.

Mom and Dad were at the computer now, in the little home office across the hall from my bedroom. Through the crack in my door I could hear them, Dad telling and retelling the events at the hospital. He was cussing a lot. I heard the office door slam shut.

I lay in my bed, shaking. I'd *never* seen Dad upset like that.

What did they just read on the computer? What did they just see?

There was no chance for sleep.

I got out of bed, put on my glasses, went to my desk, and switched on the lamp. I sat down and unzipped my backpack on the floor beside me. Whatever happened tomorrow, I knew I'd probably miss a few more weeks of school. I figured I should catch up on as much homework as I could—I needed to occupy my mind.

I decided to work on my English essay, the one about punk. I'd pretty much finished it, but I needed to proof it one last time. Miss Ray was the only cool teacher I had, anyway, so maybe she'd appreciate the effort and not load me with work while I was sick.

The title of my essay was "Punk Rock Elite." The first page touched on the history of punk—from the MC5 and the Stooges, then on to the Ramones, Sex Pistols, and the Clash. I talked about the second and third waves of punk (which is when I was introduced to it) and the way the music had changed.

But the second half of the essay—the part that I had been the most proud of—read differently to me now.

As punk rock became a successful music genre, corporations, record labels, advertising agencies, and various other sleazeballs attempted to re-create it—musically and visually—to be produced and marketed in a more profitable environment.

On many levels, this attempt was a success.

But no matter how authentic the watered-down, family-friendly version of corporate punk seems, there will always be an element lacking.

Because punk rock isn't about how fast you play, or how big your hair is; it's about attitude—a screw-you attitude that can not be manufactured, or thought up in a boardroom.

Punk is an attitude that goes beyond rebelling against disco or political parties—punk rock rebels against everything! And, oddly, I find this comforting.

Punk makes me feel like I can do anything, because the walls I see around me aren't real; religion, politics, standards, status quos—punk rock takes the power away from all those preordained establishments. It spits in the face of everything, even death.

Like the Dead Boys once sang:

> Ain't it fun
> When ya know that you're gonna die young?
> It's such fun . . .

I mean, can you imagine Avril Lavigne singing that?

That's the difference between punk rock and everything else—punk rock is a way of life.

I stared at my own words. I felt disgusted.

What a bunch of bullshit, I thought. Dying young—from

what? Self-destructive, self-obsessed crap? *Fuck that*—it doesn't count if you never see it coming.

Did any of these young punk rockers have cancer? Did any of them die slow, in a hospital gown, not a leather jacket? If they'd seen it coming, would they still have seen such romance in it? Would dying young still seem so cool?

I threw my pencil at the wall and heard it crack in the dark. I stood up and switched off the desk lamp. I was crying.

"Ain't it fun . . ." I said softly.

I cried alone, until sleep pitied me enough to show itself at last.

TEN

Die Young with Me

1

I awoke at six, like I was going to school. My eyes felt swollen as I showered. I spiked up my hair and put on my Ramones T-shirt, and then I went downstairs.

Nat was in the living room, watching TV. The coffee-maker in the kitchen hissed. It was a broken-mirror image of a normal morning, all fucked up and cracked at odd angles. The shadows fell crooked over our lives.

"You goin' to school today?" I asked Nat.

"I was going to go with y'all."

"Oh," I muttered.

I sat on the couch and stared at the TV.

"Do you not want me to go?" he asked.

I shrugged. "It isn't that, man. It just seems pointless. There's no sense for you to sit there all day—plus, Ali will feel better if she sees you at school."

"Yeah, I guess she probably would."

I handed him my English essay. He read the title out loud.

"Can you also drop that by Miss Ray's room for me?"

"How'd it turn out?"

"Like a crock of shit."

Mom hugged me as soon as she got downstairs. Dad came down behind her. He didn't say much of anything.

They both agreed that Nat should go to school—Mom promised to call the front office for him as soon as we had any news. The four of us walked out into the morning together, headed in different directions. We said a rushed goodbye, so no one had a chance to get upset.

*   *   *

"At least we'll find out where they hide the sick people," I said, forcing a laugh as we walked into the hospital.

Mom slapped my arm. We got on the elevator. Dad stared at the buttons, expressionless.

When the elevator opened, I saw my grandparents sitting in the waiting room.

"Mom," I hissed under my breath.

"Be nice," she said. "They're just worried about you."

They were dressed in their church clothes. They both hugged me, announcing that they'd come to pray for me.

Dr. Hallbeck walked into the waiting room. She hugged Mom and then she hugged me and then she hugged *everyone.* Let me tell you, when your test results are bad enough to turn your doctor into a hugger, it's a scary fucking sight.

Dr. Hallbeck walked us to the elevator and took us down to the main foyer. From there, we walked down another hallway, through the twisted spine of the building. As we walked, she explained to my parents who we were going to see, what they were going to do, until we finally arrived at Pediatric Intensive Care.

Dr. Hallbeck left us with the admitting nurse. The nurse put a hard plastic bracelet around my wrist. Another nurse came out with a clipboard and said to follow her.

She didn't check my height or weight or blood pressure—they didn't ask me any questions, they didn't even ask my name. The nurse rushed me—almost *pushed* me—into an off-white room with a bed facing a window.

She told me to get in the bed.

She took supplies out of her uniform, all wrapped in plastic. She told me to make a fist, and then stuck a long, thick needle into my hand. I yelled louder than I meant to—Mom winced.

The nurse rolled in a metal IV machine and hooked it up to the needle. Blood rose into the tube. She twisted a small knob on the plastic tube, and I watched the blood rush back into my hand and through my vein to my heart. A cold rush of clear fluid followed it in.

No one explained what was happening. No doctor had come to speak with us. Mom and Dad asked questions, but the nurses basically ignored them. One nurse taped the needle onto my hand, while the other one fucked with the keypad on the IV. It beeped like our microwave at home.

Dad wiped his eyes and left the room without a word. My grandparents followed him.

No Internet article or Bible verse could have prepared us for what was happening. There was nothing theoretical about it anymore—this was going down live, in the flesh. Our brains couldn't process it.

This isn't right, I kept thinking, *there must be some sort of mistake. Not like this. Not like this.*

One nurse brought in a bag of fluid and hung it from the top of the IV. She was about to connect it to the tube that fed into my bloodstream. Mom grabbed her with both hands and shook her.

"*Stop!*" she yelled at the nurse. "Where is the doctor? What are you about to hook up to this IV? Why haven't you done any tests? Get a doctor *NOW!*"

The nurse looked confused.

"They haven't done no tests?" the other nurse said.

"*What?*" I said.

The nurse beside Mom took my chart off the bed and looked at it. Then she looked at my plastic bracelet. Then she showed it to the other nurse. They gave each other a look and then shook their heads.

"Y'all won't believe this, but we had this boy confused with another—someone else was supposed to be in this room! Ha-ha. *Whew!*"

"I better go get a doc," the other nurse said. She left the room.

Mom was breathing as hard as I was. Her eyes were wild. She looked like she could murder both these idiots.

What the hell were they about to pump into me?

The nurse came back, holding a syringe. "The doctor is on his way," she said. She saw me looking at the syringe. "Don't worry—this is just something to help you relax."

She stuck it into the port on my hand.

I tasted chemicals—they were warm. I eased deeper into the bed.

We could've waited twenty minutes for a doctor—or it could have been all day.

I couldn't keep track of time. The drugs and the shock made everything soft. But eventually, those nurses returned with a guy in a white coat.

He introduced himself as an oncologist—a fucking cancer doctor. Dad came back into the room and stood in the corner with his arms crossed. The cancer doctor told us that I needed *specialized* care, the type they weren't able to offer in Huntington—or at any other hospital in West Virginia.

He said the hospital I had gone to didn't even have the equipment to do the type of biopsy needed—they couldn't even diagnose me, let alone treat me.

He told us that the closest hospital with the capacity to care for a case like mine was Columbus Children's Hospital, about three hours away. He'd already spoken with their head of oncology, and they were expecting me there right away.

"Ohio?" I asked weakly. My parents looked at each other.

"Okay," Mom said, "what is the next step here? Do we need to set up an appointment?"

The cancer doctor shook his head. I needed to leave right away. I needed to leave *now*. An ambulance had been arranged to transport me to Columbus as fast as possible.

"Jesus Christ, is that necessary?" Dad asked.

"More than I can even say."

I watched them all from the bed, talking about me like I wasn't there.

I sat up to walk downstairs, but a nurse eased me back into the bed. She said they'd wheel me down—like I couldn't walk myself, like I was fucking helpless. An orderly came, unlocked the brakes on my bed, and wheeled me down the hall.

My parents walked beside me, and my grandparents behind them. Mom was going to follow the ambulance to Columbus. Dad was going to ride home with Grandmother and Granddad, and then go pick up Nat. They would meet me in Columbus later that night. Dad asked if I wanted him to bring anything.

That I had the answer to: "My Minor Threat shirt. The red one. And some music."

"Anything in particular?"

"Nat will know."

They rolled me to a loading dock outside. A dark-blue ambulance was backed against the edge.

I asked if I could call Ali and tell her what was happening, but there was no time. Dad told me he loved me, and that he would see me soon. Grandmother and Granddad said a short prayer. Mom had already pulled the car around to the loading dock. She was idling there, ready to follow.

Two big EMTs lifted me off the loading dock and into the back of the ambulance. One of them walked around the front. The bigger of the two nodded at my mom, then hopped in the back with me. The ambulance bounced beneath his weight. I heard the engine start. He shut the doors.

As we pulled out of the lot, the EMT looked down at me.

"Was that you I heard asking to make a call, partner?"

"Yeah. To my girlfriend. I just wanted to tell her not to worry."

He reached into his pocket. The cell phone looked comically small in his hand.

"I know how it is," he said. "A man has *got* to check in with his woman."

He handed me the phone.

I knew that Ali wouldn't be home, but I didn't care. I didn't care if someone else heard me on the message machine either. Fuck it. The drugs had flushed all the shyness out. I waited five rings, until the message machine at her house clicked on.

"Ali. Hey. It's me. Listen, I have to go to a different hospital—a good one—in Columbus—a city hospital. I'll probably be up there for a couple days, but then I'll be back home. I just wanted to call and let you know not to worry. Everything is fine. If you need anything, call Nat. Don't worry—okay? Everything is cool. I promise."

Through the back windows of the ambulance I watched Mom follow us, keeping pace with our increasing speed. We took the same damn route my friends and I cruised on the weekends: past the park—Fifth Avenue to the viaducts—to downtown—past the buildings, straight toward the river . . .

Only this time, I was watching in reverse, through the small back windows of ambulance doors. I was watching my world be erased before my eyes.

I heard the siren sound. We were going *fast* now, blowing through red lights and blurring the cars behind us. Mom fell behind, and then she disappeared.

The ambulance shook over the cracked pavement of the Robert C. Byrd Bridge as we ran straight over the Ohio River and out the other side.

As we crossed the river, I watched my hometown fade away. The EMT injected something else into my IV line—I started nodding *in* and *out* . . .

Soon, the land was straight and flat.

We sped down an unkempt highway, past landmarks I didn't recognize. As the dead land stretched all around us, the sun appeared from behind the clouds, glaring through the windows. I could still see the river, running beside the road.

"Where does this road go?" I quietly asked the EMT.

He squinted into the light.

"Hell," he said, without looking at me. "It goes everywhere."

With the sun on my skin, I closed my eyes.

2

The last thing I remembered was arriving at the hospital in Columbus. I had fallen asleep in the ambulance (if we can refer to drug-induced unconscious episodes as sleep) and woke as I was being lifted into the air—out of the ambulance and onto the ground. The bigger EMT patted me on the shoulder.

Within seconds, two sets of hands grabbed the end of my gurney and were rolling me inside the hospital—one of them belonged to a man, the other to a woman. Both were dressed in bright purple.

I peered over the tips of my shoes as I rolled through sets of sliding doors and into a large, chaotic room. This was nothing like the hospital in Huntington. This place was *full* of people, and nothing seemed hidden—now the pain was right in front of me.

Screaming children. Parents rushing around confused and upset, trying to get answers or fill out forms or get their kid to quit crying. The tension in the room was so high, I wondered how anyone could concentrate.

Mom came through the doors behind me. She must have caught up with us somewhere outside the city. When she bent over my gurney, she looked exhausted.

A doctor approached us. He was about my dad's size, with dark, olive skin. He smiled easy.

The first thing he said was—"Man, I love that Ramones shirt!"

I knew instantly that he was something special.

He introduced himself as Mark Ranalli, the oncologist whom the Huntington doctor had spoken to. He said that they were ready for me.

While he talked to my mom about tests, purple nurses weaved around us expertly. Dr. Ranalli asked if I was still having any pain. The moment I said yes, one of the nurses moved past him and stuck a syringe in the port of my IV.

The room began to swirl around me. I felt like I was going down a drain.

"What'd you give me?" I asked the purple nurse.

"Morphine—for the pain. You try and relax now."

When she smiled, the teeth in her mouth looked blank and white and empty and then nothing.

*　*　*

But I woke up alone.

The fluorescent lights above me were dim.

Is it nighttime? There were no windows, so I couldn't say for sure. I didn't know how long I'd slept, or what day it was. All I knew was that I was alone.

I tried to sit up, but I was too weak. I rolled onto my right hip. The movement pulled the needle in my hand, ripping at the vein. I yelped like a stray dog.

I flipped onto my back again.

The movement had twisted me up in the sheets. I realized it was my hospital gown—it looked like a giant blue pillowcase. It tangled up under my armpit. I was naked underneath it.

Did I put this fucking dress on? I couldn't remember.

The thought of someone undressing me embarrassed me horribly. I thought about my gut and my drugged-up dick, flopping lamely on a gurney while some stranger pulled my jeans and underwear off as if I was a goddamn invalid.

Sometime later, Mom woke me by rubbing my shoulder, the same way she would when I didn't get up for school.

I saw her hand and nothing else; a delicate hand, with fingers a little too long for the palm. The same pale cream as my own hand, pink around the knuckles, almost translucent where blue veins pushed up against the skin. Her rings were on her fourth finger. Her nails were a bright plastic red.

I asked for my glasses—the words came out in a rasp. Mom slipped them over my ears.

This world came into focus.

Mom wore a paper medical mask over her mouth and nose. She had on the same clothes she'd worn the day we arrived at the hospital. Maybe it was the *same* day—I wasn't sure anymore. A laminated blue tag was clipped onto her shirt. It said PARENT in thick black Sharpie.

My eyeballs darted around the room. Everything was white—from the walls, to the bed, to the machines, to the computer. In the corner of the ceiling, a large white tube pumped filtered air into the room. I had my own ventilation system, separate from the rest of the hospital.

There were no windows. There was no door. One entire wall was made of thick, clear plastic. A nurse (also wearing a face mask) approached the clear wall. She put a keycard against the side and the center of the wall slid open. It sealed as soon as she entered. I felt like I was inside a fucking UFO.

"He awake now?" the nurse asked casually.

Mom nodded and kept rubbing my shoulder. The nurse took another needle and injected it into my IV. I felt warm again.

The nurse turned to go, but then questions started pouring out of my mouth uncontrollably—*Am I quarantined? Am I this contagious?*—It all came out as incoherent nonsense. There was a disconnect between mind and body, a divide that grew as the drugs spread through me . . .

. . . I floated down . . .

      . . . inside the . . .

          . . . empty space.

*   *   *

On morphine, time and memory had no place.

I existed outside myself, grasping only at random scenes from my days—things would fast-forward and rewind uncontrollably, and I watched my life projected back to me on the wall of an empty room. The film skipped, and reels were missing. There was no sound.

I was too fucked up to understand that all the precautions were to protect *me* from the outside world. "The mass" in my chest had pushed my lungs to the verge of collapse. One more week of waiting, they said, and I woulda been a goner.

I hadn't been officially diagnosed yet. Dr. Ranalli had scheduled a series of tests and was conferring with experts and specialists all over the country. Soon, they would pinpoint *exactly* what was happening inside of me and decide what—if anything—they could do about it.

The one thing that they were sure of was that the illness was extremely progressed. So they locked me in that sealed-off, germ-free room where any and all precautions would be taken until Dr. Ranalli had a game plan.

So there I was in this plastic cell. It made me think of baby pictures—of my brother and me, born premature like so many twins are. I was the smaller one, barely three pounds. We were put into incubators ironically similar to the room I was currently stuck in. I started to think that maybe I was doomed from the very start—born into a body too weak for this world.

3

These morphine-induced periods of waking unconsciousness usually included one of many daily humiliations.

It might have been my mother holding a jug to my crotch while I pissed, because I was too weak to get out of the bed. It might have been the sponge baths the male nurse gave me. Once or twice, students from the med school came by, and the room was crammed with Asian kids who looked at me like I was a science experiment.

The rest of those first days were filled with nothing but tests. Too many times a day, they did numerous tests—blood tests, biopsies, X-rays, ultrasounds, shots, scans—more medical tests than I knew existed.

Each test result led to *more* tests. Soon, I couldn't keep track of them.

I'd be fitted with a mask, and wheeled from my room to an elevator—it always went to the basement floor, into cold rooms with horrible machines. I was never sure which test I was about to endure. No matter how miserable I was in that hospital room, it was never as bad as the basement.

Most of the tests went something like this: I'd be injected with some sort of contrast, and then scanned by some giant machine. Some injections made me feel hot, some antsy, and some nauseous; but I could *always* feel the chemicals travel through my bloodstream.

Each test had its own distinctly shitty trademark.

For one scan, I was injected with a contrast that was literally radioactive—the nurse held a comically huge syringe that was encased in an inch-thick protective steel shell.

A squared-off, ominous green machine did one of the scans. It was like a demented MRI, or something— you lay inside it, and then the roof of the machine came down about a half an inch above your nose. When the scan started, the machine would *ROAR*. You couldn't move, or the results would be muddled—so you lay there for *hours*, unmoving, while the machine blasted around you. I imagine the feeling is similar to listening to the sound of a moving train (if you are tied to the tracks beneath it).

The CT scans didn't require any injections. For those, I had to *drink* the contrast—it was mixed in with a chalky red substance and masked as Kool-Aid, straight-up Jonestown style. I had to drink a certain amount every half hour. If I couldn't drink the entire container, or if I puked any of it up, I had to start the entire dose over again.

Through these tests, Dr. Ranalli was getting closer to pinpointing my condition. Clues in the scans and blood work indicated signs associated with testicular cancer, which led to a not-at-all-weird ultrasound on my balls.

From there, it led to the test I thought was the worst— the bone marrow biopsy.

I couldn't retain much from the conversations between my doctor and my parents about my condition, but I did understand that if the disease had spread into my bones (which was likely, considering the late diagnosis), then it was badterribletragic fucking news. So of all the tests, this biopsy was the one to fear.

I was made to lie on what looked like a massage table

but wasn't. Lying on my stomach made it even harder to breathe. They stuck a long, *thick* needle into my back, deep enough to suck the marrow from my spine. Goddamn, I'd never felt pain like that before (yet).

Because of all the dope, I wasn't aware enough to know that in a room similar to mine, my brother was lying face-down, waiting for his needle to drop.

Dr. Ranalli wanted to make sure Nat's body wasn't plagued with whatever biological defect was causing my illness.

Same blood, same genes, same birth, same life, same?

4

The results of the tests came back. Although it felt like weeks, the whole ordeal had actually lasted only days.

No one was expecting Dr. Ranalli when he showed up at my room. It was late in the evening, and the normally chaotic hallways of the ICU were silent. I was awake—Nat was keeping me company. He didn't mention his biopsy, or any other tests. He sat beside my bed, looking at the tubes and neon bulbs of the machines I was attached to.

The plastic wall opened and Dr. Ranalli entered, followed by my parents. They both looked utterly defeated.

Dr. Ranalli had his diagnosis.

*   *   *

I'd love to quote Dr. Ranalli's diagnosis word for word, but I can't. You see, unless you've been diagnosed with cancer, the whole process is hard to understand—everything goes completely over your head.

I used to think that cancer was a solid thing, like chicken pox or a broken neck—cancer meant you were rotting from the inside out. Cancer was a definition.

In actuality, *cancer* is more like a category—housing hundreds of diseases that can manifest in cells, blood, bones, and organs.

The medical jargon was so beyond my seventeen-year-old brain, plus the fucking drugs they kept pumping into me—I was just permanently confused, and crushed by the weight of what was happening as it was happening.

No one had ever explained to me that *mass* is a safe word for *tumor*, or that there are a hundred different ways to say *cancer*. I always thought that getting a cancer diagnosis would be more like a doctor saying, "You have cancer. Sorry, man."

But that wasn't the case.

To Dr. Ranalli and his staff, me having *cancer* was a given—they knew I had cancer as soon as they'd seen my X-ray, before I was even rolled through their doors. What he was focused on were the details of the disease—he wanted to understand its progression and, hopefully, how to cure it.

Dr. Ranalli said that I didn't have lymphoma, or leukemia. He referred to what I had as germ cell—or embryonic yolk cell—cancer. He said it was very rare.

The disease was similar to testicular cancer. Apparently, it had formed when I was a fetus—only instead of dropping with my testes, the cancer developed in the middle of my body, which explained the dark spot on my X-ray.

"So that mass . . . tumor . . . has been growing inside me . . . forever?"

Dr. Ranalli said no, not necessarily. Diagnosis often occurred in the years following puberty. He said that raging hormones are like gasoline on the infected cells.

Mom wrote down every word he said on a small yellow notepad she kept in her purse. When Dr. Ranalli was done with his explanation, she raised her hand up slightly, like a tentative student might.

"So. What happens now?"

Dr. Ranalli told us that he was working with the best team possible—and that they had a plan.

Yes—my cancer was rare. Worse—it was progressed. But the plus side was that the disease hadn't spread into my bones.

This gave Dr. Ranalli hope. And although it was anchored in my chest, the genetics of a germ cell cancer were incredibly similar to that of testicular cancer—meaning drugs that successfully treated testicular cancer might show the same results here—which is where Dr. Larry Einhorn came into the picture.

Dr. Einhorn was the head oncologist at Indiana University. He was world-renowned for his research, and most advances in the treatment of testicular cancer over the last twenty years had been due to him. He was also the personal oncologist for Lance Armstrong, who was the fucking Elvis Presley of cancer patients at the time.

Ranalli and Einhorn had been in touch since the day I arrived. Although Dr. Ranalli reached out to other experts, it was Einhorn whom he bounced every play off. Every test result that came in was discussed at length. Dr. Ranalli,

Dr. Einhorn, and their collective peers had put together an intensive treatment plan.

"How intensive?" Mom asked.

"Does it matter?" Nat said.

I was to be moved to the inpatient oncology ward, on the other side of the hospital.

My initial treatment plan consisted of six rounds of intensive chemotherapy—which would start at dawn. Each round lasted a little over a week—with a few weeks off in between for my body to recover.

Between the rounds, I would be allowed to go home.

Once the treatments began, the doses would be adjusted accordingly. If the chemotherapy worked, the tumor in my chest would shrink.

After the initial sessions, I would be sent to Indianapolis, where Dr. Einhorn and his team would remove any of the tumor that wasn't killed off by the chemo. After that, Columbus Children's would administer a few more rounds of chemo to be sure no cancerous cells remained.

Some questions from my parents followed, but not as many as you might expect.

There was little time for questions or hesitation—what my parents knew (and Nat and I didn't know) was that the disease had progressed farther along than I could've imagined. They didn't see any reason to tell me that the cancer was already Stage Four—I was lucky if I could be helped at all.

* * *

My family stuck around while we waited for an orderly to come and wheel me up to the cancer ward.

"Did Natty tell you? All your brother's tests came back negative," Dad said, trying to sound upbeat through his mask. "Thank Christ for that, at least."

He rubbed Nat on the back, but Nat shrugged Dad's arm away and stormed out through the plastic wall with his head down.

I hadn't even thought about the possibility that he could be sick—if cancer was in my cells, then *of course* he could be sick—goddamn, we shared *the same cells*. What were the chances of one of us having something this horrible, and the other one being totally fine?

Dad said good night and went off to find Nat. The two of them were headed back to the hotel. I sat there trying to process what I'd heard.

How would I feel if it was the other way around, I wondered. *Guilty? Lucky? Both?*

Probably all of those things, but I knew that Nat didn't *want* to be lucky—not if I wasn't. He wouldn't want to be out there alone. He was with me there in the bcfore; he would be with me in the after.

* * *

The orderly was a skinny black kid with a set of headphones around his neck. He pushed my wheelchair into the staff elevator and pressed 6—up to the cancer ward.

The elevator opened. The walls were purple, just like the nurses' uniforms. There were two heavy doors ahead. Sheets of clear plastic hung from the corner wall.

"Sorry about the mess," he said. "They're doin' lots of renovation up here. But hey, hopefully you won't be around to see it finished."

He pressed a button and waited to be let into the ward.

"I mean, you know—like, you 'won't be around' 'cause you're *cured*. I didn't mean that you'd be dead, or nothing, you know?"

The doors opened onto a pure white hallway. Mom was already there, introducing herself at the nurses' station.

"We're in room seven," she said.

He wheeled me down the hall and she followed behind us. Every door we passed was closed.

Room seven was twice as big as the spaceship room. There was a window where I could see traffic lights and rooftops. There was a bed, a chair, a TV, and a bathroom.

A nurse got my IV situated. She and my mom helped me into the bed. Then she left the two of us alone.

The room was a soft teal color, with bright yellow fish painted on one wall.

"This room looks like a fucking day care," I said.

Mom laughed. She came over to the bed and removed my glasses for me.

"Honey, it's a *children's* hospital—what do you expect?"

I rolled my eyes.

Mom dimmed the lights and stretched out in the chair.

"I'm gonna pass out soon, Mom. You can go ahead back to the hotel y'all are staying at."

"I'm not going to leave you here by yourself—this chair is comfortable. I'm fine right here."

I didn't say anything back. I just lay there, in the stiff

bed of my cold hospital room, trying to relax. It was easier with her beside me. Some people need guardian angels. I had my mom.

5

When I woke up, Mom was gone.

The sun was shining outside; the light slashed bright stripes across my blanket through the blinds. For the first time since my arrival, I felt like I was awake.

In the corner, a janitor was holding the unused waste-basket over a trash bag. He peered inside of it—paused— and then dumped it over the bag anyway.

I propped myself up on my elbows and cleared my throat. He sat the trash can down loudly.

"Look who's up," he said. "Welcome, Youngblood."

"Hey."

He moved around the edges of the room, searching for things to pick up.

"If you're looking for your mamma, she's down at the bathroom by the end of the hall."

"Oh, thanks."

I lay back down and closed my eyes. The janitor ran his hands through the plastic cushions of the chair, still speaking

"The nurses got a kick out of *her*, boy. Did you know one of the late-shift girls told your mamma that visiting hours were over, and she had to leave?"

"No."

"You know what she told that nurse?"

"What?"

"She told her to get bent!" he said, bursting into laughter.

"Sounds about right."

He walked into the hallway and came back with a mop.

"The other nurses can't quit laughing about it," he said. "But it *worked*—didn't it? So more power to her."

"Guess so."

"They were talkin' about you too. You're some rock star, huh?"

"Not exactly."

"*Sheeeiiit*, I heard our new boy was the *real* deal—heard him and his brother had some traveling rock 'n' roll group. I must have the wrong room."

"It's *punk*," I said, coughing. "It isn't a rock 'n' roll band, it's punk rock."

The janitor laughed again.

"I've known some sorry-ass punks in my day, but I got a feeling you ain't one of them."

I looked at the tube running into my arm.

"Guess we'll see," I mumbled.

He mopped the bathroom and walked back into the hall. He posted on the open door, nodding toward me.

"You ain't no punk, kid. I know you're probably scared as hell. But that will pass. You just gotta hang tough."

"Thanks. I'm trying."

"*Trust* me, Youngblood—if you're anything like your mamma, you gonna be all right."

* * *

A few minutes later, a nurse took a blood sample. She couldn't take it from the same arm that the IV was in, so a new needle got stuck in my opposite arm—test tube after test tube filled thick with dark red—it was a hell of a way to wake up.

"Time for your medicine," she said.

One by one, she dropped pills out of a Dixie cup and into my hand. I counted seven total; different sizes and shapes, all equally unfamiliar to me—I swallowed them all without question.

When Mom came back she wore the same clothes but had applied a fresh coat of makeup. An orderly came in with breakfast, while we watched some dumb story about Tom Cruise on the *Today* show.

I couldn't remember the last time I ate. But when Mom removed the lid—scrambled eggs—the way the grease mixed with the bleach smell of the hospital made me grimace.

"I can't eat this crap," I said. "I don't wanna puke."

I hadn't talked to Ali since I was admitted. Nat had been giving her updates, so at least she knew I'd been too sick to talk. Mom mentioned that Nat was thinking about bringing her up to visit me over the weekend—if I was up to it.

I groaned in reply, dreading the thought of anyone seeing me this way.

A few hours later, the door opened again. A woman walked in. She was young, maybe in her twenties, and the tallest chick I'd ever seen. Her legs stretched up and up and up, up under her white lab coat, up all the way to her golden-blond hair.

She greeted me excitedly, explaining that we'd met

when I was too drugged up to remember. She reintroduced herself—Stacey Whiteside, Dr. Ranalli's nurse practitioner.

"You can't be a nurse," I said. "You aren't wearing one of those ugly purple getups."

Stacey laughed. "A nurse practitioner is kind of a half nurse, half doctor—and the biggest perk is that I can skip the purple."

"Right on," I said. I tried to smile.

Stacey had come by to tell us that it was time for me to start chemotherapy. She went over the drugs that would be administered—cisplatin, bleomycin, and something called VP16.

Things were getting way too real. I was nervous.

Is my hair gonna fall out?—"Most patients do temporarily lose it. But not all."

How long does it take?—"Each dose takes five to eight hours to complete."

Am I going to puke?—"Definitely."

Stacey also said the chemo could make me feel very weak. "Because of your age," she added, "we want to make sure we're giving you the right dosage. Different ratios are used for children and adults—and you fall right in between. Teenagers always make life *so* much more complicated. . . ."

When it was time for my chemotherapy to actually begin, they let me sit in the chair instead of the bed. Two nurses came in. One connected three new, full bags of chemicals to the top of my IV. The other took the trash can from the corner and sat it beside my chair.

"Are you ready?" the nurse said.

"I guess."

She pressed the keypad on the IV. I watched a little bubble make its way from one of the chemo bags slowly, through the IV, into the needle, and then inside of me. I was determined not to puke.

I'd made up my mind. No matter how nauseous I felt, there was no fucking way I was going to puke (*if I can stop myself from puking, maybe I can stop my hair from falling out*). The drugs affected everyone differently—Stacey said so herself. For once in my life, I was determined to land on the winning end of a spectrum.

Five minutes—nothing.

Mom asked if I needed anything. I didn't reply. I sat stoically, concentrating on nothingness.

Seven minutes—I felt *odd*.

This wasn't nausea. I didn't know what the hell this was.

Sixteen minutes—I was struggling.

A weird, uncomfortable warmth ran through my entire body, all pinpointed at my stomach and throat. I tensed all my neck muscles, trying to shut off my gag reflex.

Don't think about it don't think about it don't think about it don't.

Sixteen and a half minutes—I puked my fucking guts out.

*　　*　　*

Nausea and vomiting take on different meanings for chemo patients. You can't think of these words in a normal context. Even food poisoning doesn't come close to the sickness that chemotherapy drugs bring on—for that, you have to be poisoned by something much more dangerous than gas station sushi. Something powerful, something *radioactive*. Maybe even something fatal.

Because that's what I was doing—poisoning myself.

It's some kind of *Twilight Zone* episode, where you have to kill yourself to save your own life. The cells you destroy are *your* cells. So when they pump those drugs into your system, your system knows they shouldn't be there and it freaks the fuck out.

Unlike normal vomiting, puking during chemo offers no relief. You can't purge yourself of the horrible things inside you.

All you can do is try to get through it.

I puked for *hours*.

The stuff that came out of my body had the colors and smell of a chemical disaster. It wasn't human.

If I tried to speak, I puked. If I smelled the puke, I puked. If I puked on myself, I puked at the sight. The more I puked, the more I puked. I puked when there was nothing *to* puke, dry-heaving spit and pinkish chemical bile.

The IV bags were empty, but I kept puking. It wouldn't let up.

I sat in my chair and kept my head down. A nurse asked if I needed to go to the bathroom. I stood up but was too weak to walk. Mom and the nurse helped me back into bed. The nurse went into the hall to find another plastic piss bottle.

Soon after, an orderly brought in a tray—dinner. I puked before he had a chance to open the lid.

I lay on the bed, lifeless. A different nurse came with pills and water.

She sat them on the side table. I grunted at her. She said to be careful not to throw up the pills.

Why can't you just inject me with pills? You inject me with everything else under the motherfucking sun.

One at a time, Mom held the pills up to my lips—until I had no choice but to swallow. By the time the nurse came back, the pills were gone. She took my blood again, and then injected my IV with something to help me sleep.

She came back one last time—with a pillow and extra blankets for Mom.

Mom thanked her and flipped off the light. The room was cast in fluorescent afterglow. Then it grew dark, the machines beeping low like a pulse.

My first day of treatment was done.

6

Nat sat with me the next day, while Mom showered at their hotel. He brought me some clothes, but they wouldn't let me change out of my gown. It was total bullshit.

A nurse came to the door with a wheelchair. She said our parents were down in the cafeteria, with a pizza.

"Jesus Christ," I said, frustrated. "She *knows* I can't eat that stuff."

"It's cool," Nat told the nurse. "I'll wheel him. I know the way."

Nat wheeled me down the hall of the ward, past the other hospital rooms. Again, all of the doors were shut. We took the elevator to the lobby that led to the cafeteria. The nurse made me wear a protective face mask.

It was the first time I'd seen the front lobby of the hospital. The walls were bright colors; the carpet was (you guessed it) purple. The whole place seemed cluttered, like a child's playroom—which it kind of was.

Rolling through the lobby and seeing all those kids just felt *weird*—some of them were obviously serious cases. Some of them were crippled. But they all seemed oblivious to it. They were running around, playing, climbing, crying—all the stuff that normal little kids do. Their parents sat far away from each other, watching the children with heartbroken eyes.

I related more to the parents than to the kids.

I didn't feel oblivious. I understood the gravity of my situation. I mean, think about it—I was *almost* eighteen. I had driven a car, I had seen a girl naked (in person), I knew shitloads of cusswords—but here I was, stuck at the stupid kids' table.

"I gotta ask, bro," Nat said. "What the fuck is up with all the purple?"

I just sighed.

"I know Mom can be annoying, but you've got to eat, dude—you know you do."

"Fuck that."

"Whatever. You know that you haven't eaten in four

days, right? Actually, fuck it—don't eat. At least you're finally getting skinny."

"It's the chemo," I said. "I can't even *talk* about food without feeling sick."

"So eat! What's the big deal? You're gonna puke it up, anyway."

"Good point, I guess."

He kept making small talk, but I zoned out. I wanted to talk to him—about the band, about Ali, about us—but I just couldn't do it. I had to put the little energy I had toward not throwing up inside of my face mask.

The air in the lobby was stifling. It was deodorized with bleach and chemicals and who knows what—just like the rest of the waiting rooms. They always wanted to hide the smell of *sick*, keep it locked up on the top floors so visitors didn't have to think about it. But I could smell it now.

I just didn't realize the smell was coming from me.

7

"I heard you got some friends coming today," the janitor said. He had his work cut out for him now—with the puke and shit and the smell of drug-sweat.

"Yep," I said. "My girlfriend too."

"There ya go, I know how you rock stars do," he said, and winked.

I laughed a lot when he was around, no matter how bad I felt. The janitor never asked my name, and I never asked his. But it was amazing how good it felt to get treated like a normal dude, if only for a few minutes.

When the morning shift nurse drew my blood, she told me that I was allowed to take a bath. Not a sponge bath—a *real* bath, my first since I'd arrived.

She ran the bathwater for me. When it was ready, she helped me into my bathroom. The bathtub had two support rails around it, and a call switch on the wall. She wrapped my IV port in sandwich wrap so it wouldn't get wet. I told her that I could take my own gown off. Tentatively, the nurse left me alone in the bathroom. I eased into the water, trying not to slip. It felt amazing. I felt almost human again.

Damn, I really am getting skinny.

For the first time in my life, my stomach looked flat. Not in a good way, exactly, but screw it. I couldn't believe I'd puked *that* much.

I used the crappy soap bar, and I had a plastic cup to rinse with. As I washed my chest, I saw the soap get covered in hair. I looked at my washcloth—it was full of little dark hairs too. I scanned my body, but saw no big clumps missing. I looked at the washcloth again.

I ran my hand onto my chest and pulled at a hair. Then I pulled some more. Then I did the same thing to my head . . . *Fuckfuckfuck.* They came out easily, with no sensation at all. I was pulling dead leaves from a tree.

There was a knock at the door—it was the nurse.

"I have a new gown for you. Cover your privates with the washcloth and I will come help you out."

I did as I was told, wondering how much pride I had left to lose.

*　　*　　*

Nat walked my friends up to the ward.

When he knocked, I was positioned in my chair (the bed would have been way too dramatic). I psyched myself up to act as normal as possible, even though all I really felt like doing was sleeping.

But I have to say, as soon as my friends walked in I felt a hundred times better. Nat came in first—Paul, Ashley, and Brody followed. They moved around the room carefully, like they were trying to avoid some trapdoor that we'd all already fallen through.

Then Ali walked in.

She looked like a daydream. She wore more makeup than usual—her eyes were outlined in thick mascara that seemed way too sexy for a hospital visit. If the sight of me troubled her, she didn't let it show.

She had her arms around me before I could even stand up.

We didn't talk about my condition, or any of that depressing shit. We talked about the same stuff we would talk about anywhere, the bullshit teen crap that kids talk about in school hallways, or on the phone late at night. Goddamn, I'd missed it.

Paul had a camera with him and kept taking snapshots of us all. Ashley and Nat sat on the corner of the bed, and Ali sat on the floor by my side. Brody had a backpack full of stuff that they'd brought me.

He handed me a shoe box full of handmade GET WELL cards. I began sorting through them. I was touched that so many people had gone to the trouble, but I saw that only a few cards were from my friends—most of the names I didn't even recognize.

Slowly, I realized that they were all from kids in my fifth-period Spanish class. *It was for school credit? Jesus.*

I put the box away.

Next, Brody pulled out a stack of porno. It musta been a foot high. On top of the smut pile was a *Penthouse* with Briana Banks on the cover. She looked like she could eat me alive.

"Ha-ha! Thanks, man. But you know I like chicks with dark hair," I said, and squeezed Ali's hand.

I put the magazines away for later inspection.

Ali brought me a small cross, and a prayer card with the Archangel on it. I wasn't religious—but when you date a Catholic you can't help getting a little on you. The cross was small and silver. Not a fancy thing, squared off on the ends. Engraved on it was:

<pre>
        J
        E
L O V E S Y O U
        U
        S
</pre>

"Thanks, baby."

"You promise you like it?" she asked.

"Goddamn right I do."

She nodded. She found some medical tape in a drawer and taped the little cross to my bedrail. She told me to look at it every night.

"At least he'll be safe from vampires," Brody said.

Everyone but Ali laughed.

"Show him the magazine," Ashley said softly.

Nat and Brody looked at each other and grinned. Slowly, Brody pulled a copy of *Rolling Stone* out of his backpack. He tossed it in my lap.

"Turn to page one twenty-eight," Nat said.

I flipped through the magazine until I got to a two-page article titled "Punks Rejoice—Warped Tour '01 Announces Official Lineup." I scanned through the article, faster and faster, skipping the bullshit—near the end there was a full listing of bands: 311, Good Charlotte, Dropkick Murphys, AFI, Flogging Molly, Jimmy Eat World, the Distillers . . . Defiance of Authority . . .

My jaw fucking dropped—we were in *Rolling* fucking *Stone*! *WHAT?!?!*

"Dude!" I yelled. "Holy shit!"

"I know!"

"I mean *shit*!"

"I know!"

My eyes kept drifting to the *Rolling Stone*.

Seeing our name in print was the most validating thing that had ever happened to me. But I could only imagine how Nat and Brody felt, even Paul must have wondered what the hell we were going to do now that I was in the hospital. No one had mentioned it, but we all knew it needed to be dealt with—*now*.

I felt like I'd blown it for everyone. Our band would never get a chance like this again. Not kids like us. Not in West Virginia.

"Look, guys," I said, leaning forward. "I think we are gonna have to find a fill-in drummer for the tour."

"Fuck *that*," Nat said instantly.

No one else said anything.

"You were in here when the doc went over my treatment plan," I said to him. "I don't think I'll even be done with chemo by the summer—it makes me so fucking weak, bro, there's no way."

"Maybe your doctors can schedule treatments around the shows. Push them back a week or something."

"I don't think it works like that," Brody said.

"Really?" Nat snapped. "How the fuck would *you* know how it works?"

I sighed. "It wouldn't matter, anyway. Even if they were willing to do that . . . y'all just don't understand how shitty I feel. I can barely get into the bathroom—how am I gonna go on tour?" I held up the magazine. "There is *no way* I want to fuck this up any more than I already have—you guys *have* to do the tour. *You have to*."

"Who would you want to fill in?" Paul asked.

"I haven't given it much thought."

"I have a few ideas," Brody said, "I'll put some feelers out . . . if you want me to . . . and then we can start auditioning. Any of the drummers around town would kill to do it."

"We need to wait until Rob is home before we try anyone out," Nat said. "*Rob* is going to pick the fill-in. It's his band as much as anyone's."

"Wouldn't have it any other way," Brody said.

Nat ran his hand through his hair. "But for the record, I think this fucking sucks."

* * *

There was one more item inside the backpack—clippers. Paul had been shaving his head for years. At home, I never woulda considered cutting my hair off. My fucking hair was my best feature. But after seeing those pathetic hairs matted to my washcloth, I suddenly thought it was a great idea. Maybe I was still in shock.

I instructed Ali on how to help me walk my IV into the bathroom. The towel from my bath was on the floor, and she wrapped it around my neck. Paul flipped on his clippers, and I leaned over the sink.

"I always knew you wanted to jock my style," he said.

I felt the vibrations run over my skull. My hair was pretty thick, and still covered in clumps of glue, so it took five passes to shear through it. I stared into the sink, watching bleached hairs rain down. When Paul turned off the clippers, my ears were ringing.

I looked up at the mirror and I saw a different person.

Without hair, I *did* look thin. My head shrank back behind my glasses. I wasn't totally bald—I had a head full of stubble, just like Paul. I could see his reflection as he admired his work.

"Now *that's* a hell of a haircut," he said.

Ali rubbed the hair off my neck and shoulders. She said she loved it. Nat said that I looked like Dad. I checked my reflection again.

Mom came into the room. She didn't seem surprised by my haircut. She walked over and rubbed the stubble.

"I wanted to come tell you it's almost time for your treatment," she said.

The room got quiet. I couldn't let them stay while I got chemo, not even Nat. I told everyone that it was time to go.

We said our goodbyes and made plans for home—shit to do, movies to see, the normal stuff. No one had the energy to talk about the band anymore.

Finally, they left—everyone but Ali. Nat shut the door to give us some privacy.

We sat beside each other on my bed, holding hands like we did on our first date. She was careful not to twist my IV port.

She asked me if I hurt. I lied and said no. I wrapped my arm around her waist and held her as tight as my weak body would let me.

But soon, she was gone. Replaced by the nurse, strapping those bags of poison up again.

*　*　*

As I was going to sleep that night, I looked at the cross now taped to my bed. It seemed wrong to start believing in God just because I was sick—how many people had done the exact same shit, in the exact same bed?

It wasn't like I *didn't* believe, anyway. I'd simply never cared. But there I was, staring at a hospital cross.

Fuck it, I thought.

I shut my eyes.

God, I prayed silently, *listen—if you let me survive, I'll do* anything. *Straight up—I'll be a good dude. I swear. I'll stop listening to Bad Religion and Agnostic Front. I'll quit saying "goddamn" all the time. Anything.*

Please—just don't let me die, God. Please just let me get out of here, just let me live. You've gotta fucking let me live—I will make good. I swear.

Amen.

With that, I fell asleep quickly—feeling safe in the knowledge that neither of us would let the other one down.

8

The day after my friends left, Dad and Nat did too. Dad came down with a cold, so he was no longer allowed on the ward. Besides, my parents wanted Nat back in school. They had to call my room to tell me goodbye.

Tom Petty once sang that days went by like paper in the wind. That was exactly how it felt in the hospital. I was living in a time zone all to myself—hours moved all around me, sometimes slowly, but sometimes blowing away so quickly that I barely noticed them pass.

The drugs played a big part, but it was more than that; Mom and I had eased into a routine. A sick routine that I hate to even think about—wake, blood, pills, puke, shit, puke, sleep, puke, pills, blood, drugs, pray, sleep.

But the humiliations and tests were not the only thing that broke up the monotony—sometimes I got random visitors: a clown, a comfort dog, a football player doing a photo op. A therapist came by a few times, but I wasn't into it. Once, a priest stopped by. He left me a copy of the New Testament—a picture Bible for kids. I put it in the pile with Briana and the girls.

When my final day of chemo arrived, it felt like forever, and no time at all.

The morning after my last injection, I woke to the never-ending headache of being processed out of the hospital. I spent the first half of the day going through the now-familiar list of tests and scans. A dietician came by a few hours later with a stack of printed-out dietary restrictions and suggestions. The printouts said I needed to eat at least five thousand calories a day. She told me to drink Ensure, like a grandmother. . . .

I nodded—*yes, ma'am*—I'd do whatever I needed to, so long as they let me leave.

Stacey came to see me. She had papers too—a giant list of prescriptions. She went over all of them, how to take them, when to take them, on and on. She warned me about possible mouth sores and prescribed some chemical rinse to prevent them. I barely paid attention. I was sure Mom would remember it all.

Stacey hung around the room until Dr. Ranalli came by.

He said the discharge papers were almost processed. He started warning us to keep an eye out for new side effects—I yawned. Once I left the hospital, I'd feel fine. I wouldn't be getting dosed with poison. I couldn't imagine the side effects following me home.

When Dr. Ranalli was leaving, Mom hugged him for a really long time. He turned around as he left my room and yelled, *"And NO skateboarding!"*

He laughed into the hallway. Stacey gave us both

(lucky me) hugs, and said to call if we noticed any more side effects.

By the time the nurse brought in my paperwork, it was nearly eight at night. But I couldn't bitch about it—I couldn't bitch about *anything*—I was going home.

She unhooked me from the IV but then inserted a temporary port into my bicep—one needle slid out, another slid in. She promised that it would mean less shots for my blood work. All it meant to me was that there was a four-inch tube dangling off my damn arm. The nurse curled it and wrapped tape around it.

When Mom pulled out a set of clothes that Nat had brought me, I started to get stoked. Goddamn—I mean, goshdarn—I'd never wanted to feel *normal* so bad in my life!

The clothes hung off me, literally.

My Minor Threat shirt looked oversize, and my pants hung from my ass even worse than usual. *I must have lost twenty pounds,* I thought. Actually, I'd lost twenty-three.

"They're here with the wheelchair," Mom said.

I kept staring at myself in the bathroom mirror.

"Cool. Let's go home."

* * *

If there were sights on the way out of town, it was too dark to see them.

All I saw was traffic, and the shadows of buildings. The on-ramp of the interstate was jammed with cars; horns and headlights surrounded us and made my head throb.

But once we got off the interstate things were quiet, and Mom promised US-23 ran all the way home.

The land outside the city was flat and empty, just like I remembered. No neighborhoods, just random homes with barren acres of land separating them. It was the kind of dark that only exists in the in-between.

There were no other cars on the road. Our headlights stretched out for miles. In the rearview mirror I watched the road, lit red by our taillights, fade back into the black, empty night.

Somewhere outside Chillicothe the clouds let go of the moon, and dull yellow patches appeared in the sky. I looked out the window—there was the moon again, reflecting off water running just yards from the road.

"Is that our river?" I asked.

It was.

*   *   *

I fell asleep sometime after that. When Mom woke me, the car was no longer moving. I looked around and yawned. It took me a moment to realize I was home—we were parked beneath the oak trees in front of our house.

Mom was already out of the car, pulling her things from the trunk. I unbuckled my seat belt but hesitated. I looked toward the house.

The lights were on downstairs, the same comfortable yellow as the moon on the river. But I just couldn't shake the feeling they were burning for someone else.

SIDE B

Broken bodies in a death rock dance hall,
Please be my partner. . . .

—The Misfits
("All Hell Breaks Loose")

ELEVEN

Half In/Half Out

1

I woke to the sound of birds, talking in the way that birds talk. I heard a car skid as it bounced over the cracked bricks on our road. My sheets felt heavy and warm.

I opened my eyes.

There was no janitor. No tubes, no beeping. I reached for my glasses—*there*, on the side table. I put them on. I sat up.

I looked around my old bedroom. *My* posters. *My* skateboard. *My* stereo. *My* dirty laundry on the floor—the whole fucking room was untouched.

I looked at *my* alarm clock. Red lights spelled 12:42. I groaned and got out of bed. I walked slowly into *my* bathroom and pissed in *my* toilet—no IV, no piss bottle or nurse or mom. I smiled.

Damn, it was good to be home.

I walked downstairs. I walked through the house. It was quiet.

I saw a cluster of pill vials sitting on the kitchen

173

counter—dozens of them, sitting out in the open like we were running some goshdarn methadone clinic.

I found Mom in the backyard, reading in her chipped white wicker chair. I sat down on the back stairs and looked up at the clouds. The lukewarm late-April breeze gave me gooseflesh. I breathed in the smell of grass and young flowers, remembering what it meant to have the sun on my skin.

Mom called to me. She said I wasn't allowed in direct sunlight without sunblock—doctor's orders, like I could die of melanoma after five minutes of fresh air.

* * *

I took my first shower in almost two weeks. Mom helped me wrap a trash bag over the port in my upper arm. She asked me to leave the bathroom door unlocked.

I turned the HOT knob as far right as it would go. I leaned my head against the tile and sucked in the heat. The steam and the water rinsed the debris from my body and the bad thoughts from my mind. I stayed in there until the hot water ran out.

Out of the shower, my body looked as sleek as a pale pink wet suit. My chest hair was gone now. Puberty in reverse. I whipped the steam from the mirror and squinted at myself—I realized that my eyebrows were almost gone too. It gave me an expressionless appearance. I almost didn't look human.

I spent the better part of an hour getting dressed, enjoying getting to wear something besides a backless gown. I threw on an old Zero Skateboards long-sleeve. I reached for my jacket—but then remembered it was the one I wore on the day of my X-ray. I put it back on the rack. I never touched it again.

I grabbed a black beanie from my bottom drawer. I pulled it down on my head as far as it would go, until the threads reached the top of my glasses—a temporary fix to my eyebrow problem.

When I walked back downstairs, Nat and Paul were sitting in the living room. They said we were going to go out to the Pizza Buffet, the way we sometimes used to. I tried to act energetic and followed them out to the van.

Man, I'd missed our van. Our smelly, ugly fucking van. I missed the cigarette holes in the seats and the crack in the windshield. I missed all of it.

Nat picked up our buddy Tyson first. I hadn't seen him since before I got diagnosed, but when he climbed into the backseat he did his best not to act shocked by my change in appearance. He told me that I looked good.

Then Nat drove to Ali's house. Paul walked with me up to her front door.

When the door swung open, Ali was wearing my old Descendents shirt. Add that to her tight jeans and eye makeup, and she almost looked punk.

She squeezed me. The curves of her body moved against mine. I sighed.

"Okay, lovebirds," Paul said, "Let's go get fucking pizza before y'all make me lose my appetite."

Nat parked at the very end of the Pizza Buffet parking lot. We got out of the van and walked toward the restaurant. A few yards from the door, I stopped.

I looked down for a moment—and then projectile vomited all over the blacktop. The puke was thick and bright pink, chewed bubble gum mixed with roadkill guts. It poured out of me in one heavy stream.

My friends stood in shock, covering their mouths. They backed away from me. The puke kept coming. A pink, chunky pile of it seeped across the parking lot. I felt it soak into my shoes.

Pizza Buffet customers watched from the restaurant window. After an eternity of puking, the manager came out to see what was happening. He saw me and cringed.

"What are you doing to our lot?" he yelled.

"You got a fucking problem?" Nat said.

"Go the fuck back inside!" Paul yelled.

The manager walked backward, toward the door.

"Don't even *look* at him, asshole," Nat said, "or he is gonna puke all over *you* next! Then he is going to go inside and puke all over this shitty pizza!"

The manager adiosed.

I wiped off my mouth, panting. I looked down at the mess.

"Well," I said, "thanks for lunch."

*   *   *

I mostly stayed home after that.

I was bummed—I'd thought that the puking and sickness would only happen *during* the chemo sessions, not in between them. But damn, was I wrong. I felt nauseous constantly.

But all in all, my life out of the hospital wasn't much different from how I was before I went in.

I was still sick, but it was a different kind of sick.

I spent a lot of time sitting on the front porch. It was a safe distance from the bathroom, and if I couldn't make it Dad would hose the mess off the concrete. I could stay out of the sun but still be out in the world.

I rocked in our old green swing, looking over at the houses and colored mailboxes. I admired the way the yards rolled down through the oaks and over the bumpy brick street. I traced the houses *up*, over their gutters and roofs and chimneys, out to the green hills that rose at their backs.

With every day that passed, each sunset seemed a little less like a mirage.

2

The side effects felt different than they did in the hospital. I wasn't sure if the changes were manifesting, or if they'd been present ever since I started treatment and I'd just been too sick to know. But now that I was free from the physical/mental wasteland of chemotherapy, I was beginning to notice a lot of weird shit.

For instance—I was finally getting my appetite back. In fact, now that I was home I felt hungry all the time. But food tasted terrible. Fucking *inedible*.

It was insane—the drugs had ruined my taste buds.

Now, anything sweet tasted sickly syrupy. Anything dairy tasted spoiled. *Everything* good tasted *bad*. My mouth felt dirty all the time.

I had two separate chemical washes to prevent the mouth sores that are common in association with cancer treatments. I swished them around my mouth three times a day—they had the aftertaste of a hospital room.

After a few days back, I wasn't puking *as much* as I did while receiving chemo. But nausea started appearing in other forms. Mainly debilitating diarrhea. Just when I'd thought life couldn't get more disgusting, it did—the strange sights and smells that came from my body were like something from the refinery that sat on the outside of town.

I was stuck in the bathroom for hours on end, my stomach cramped into knots no medicine could untie. Sometimes, I was so full of this chemical waste I'd be puking and shitting at once, an act that defied nature and everything good and reasonable in this gross, fucked-up world.

Even more constant than the nausea was a strange tingling in my hands and feet—it was an odd, constant sting, as if my limbs were asleep. The constant tingling made it hard for me to grip. I dropped glasses and plates, and sometimes my hand slipped while opening doors.

Mom called Stacey about it. She said it was likely nerve damage from the bleomycin. To dull the effects, she prescribed me three more pills.

Although I felt more coherent than I had in the hospital, I started experiencing what is referred to as "chemo brain" (the stupid name makes light of how shitty it really is). My thoughts kept getting scrambled up, like my circuits weren't firing in time. I'd forget what I was saying mid-sentence, and would sometimes switch thoughts and conversations seamlessly, and without reason.

The toxicity of the chemotherapy drugs also caused tinnitus, a constant ringing in my ears—a swirling, steady hum, as if I was living inside a seashell.

I remember the first time I noticed it. I was standing on the porch, talking to Paul—but I couldn't make out what he was saying. My ears were ringing as if I'd just left the front row of a loud concert.

I moved closer. I asked Paul to repeat himself. But all I could concentrate on was the *hummmmmmmmm*.

The tinnitus started driving me crazy. It was fucking horrible. Even with the drugs and exhaustion, the ringing in my ears made it hard to sleep. It became even harder to concentrate. Sometimes I could barely think.

The only way I could ignore the ringing in my ears was to concentrate on something else. It had to be something that I could set on a loop—a constant to negate a constant. It had to be something that could be in my every thought without driving me fucking insane.

It had to be music.

So I played music in my head constantly. It was usually just a verse, or a single riff dubbed over the hum and set on repeat. I sectioned my consciousness into two parts— one of them inward and constant, the other struggling to keep a grasp on the world around me.

I pulled it off pretty good, as long as you didn't mind that I began every conversation with the words "Um . . . huh?"

There were pills for side effects and pills for breathing. There were pills that seemed just for the sake of it. Some pills were so large, Mom had to cut them up with a steak knife.

I took them all diligently—*give me ALL the pills*—even as my regimen stretched to twenty-seven different pills a day. But none of them helped relieve the ringing in my ears, the exhaustion in my bones, or the sunspots on my brain.

I just swallowed them down and wished for the best.

3

After a week at home, I had to go all the way to Columbus just to get my blood drawn. It sounds ridiculous, but after my experience at the hospital in Huntington, Dr. Ranalli didn't want them involved in my care.

Going back to Children's Hospital was surprisingly anticlimactic. I didn't see Dr. Ranalli or Stacey. I didn't even have to go to the cancer ward.

I just had to see a nurse, get some blood drawn, and get slapped with a Batman Band-Aid. We were only there about forty minutes, and then we were back on the road for the long drive home.

It was the drive that bothered me.

The sky was gray. The barren landscape was a drag—it stretched out three hours long. Such a long drive for such a short trip.

The time seemed wasted.

I only had a week left. A week at home, and then I'd

be back on this road, on my way to have poison pumped back in my veins.

*   *   *

I got a letter in the mail from my cousin Anthony, post-marked from Richmond, Virginia.

I hadn't heard from him in years. I tore the envelope open. There was a card inside with a cartoon cat wearing sunglasses. *Stay Cool, Cat*, the cartoon said. I rolled my eyes and opened the card.

Hey dude, hope you start feeling better soon. Heard you guys are going on tour! HELL YES! Living the fucking dream, dude! Do EVERYTHING that I would do. I know you will. You got that fucked-up Rufus Blood running through those veins.

STAY UP—Anthony.

It made me a little sad. He talked about the tour like I was still going. But whatever, I had to smile. He knew our band was on the tour, didn't he?

He knew that we weren't posers, after all.

That same day, Nat brought home the term paper I'd written about punk rock. There was an A+ and a smi-ley face drawn in the corner. On the back of the paper, Miss Ray had written a long note—she wrote a lot of nice things, things that most teachers wouldn't say to some shy kid who sat in the back and never raised his hand.

I remember that note so well, because I didn't hear from any of my other teachers ever again.

The school year was ending in about a month, so our principal told my parents that the school would pass me for the semester with whatever my GPA was before I "left." All of my teachers had agreed to the idea, except one. My first-period biology teacher said that if I didn't do the final project—dissecting a pig—it would constitute an automatic F.

The thought of a science teacher being so flippant about a student's cancer diagnosis was something I couldn't compute. What did he care if I dissected a dead pig? It wouldn't affect him either way. Was the old bastard *that* jaded on life?

Fuck it, I thought, *my hands are so numb I can barely hold a fork. How am I supposed to cut the guts out of a dead animal? If he wants to fail me for being sick, let him fail me.*

So he did.

4

I hadn't had any "alone time" with Ali ever since I got home from the hospital. Anytime I wanted to kiss her, I became self-conscious about the sores in my mouth. And I couldn't imagine that she'd want to kiss me in this state.

I knew that I looked different—bald, gross, sick. Some days, I felt like it wasn't so bad. *Most* days, my reflection made me feel like I was looking at a walking corpse.

But no matter how bad I felt—physically or mentally—I still wanted her.

She was dressing more punk every day. She was caking on the eyeliner. As the temperature rose, her outfits shrank. Apparently, my libido was the only thing strong enough to survive the effects of the cancer treatments.

So when Ali's parents left town on the Friday before

I went back to Columbus, I figured it was my chance to get her alone. But when I called her, she told me that she was having a small party—just a few friends. She asked me if I wanted to come. Normally, I would have said no. But my chances of getting laid were better with a house full of friends than they were with a house full of parents, *sooooo*—I told her I'd see her there.

Mom and Dad made me promise that I wouldn't drive alone. They were worried I would get too tired. I asked Nat to go, but he had plans with Ashley. So I called Paul— he told me to meet him outside in ten.

I tossed my nighttime dose of pills into the little metal pill carrier that Mom bought me. I stuffed it into my pocket, beside my breath mints.

When Paul and I pulled off Forrest Road and into Ali's driveway, there were nearly a dozen cars parked off the shoulder. Paul pulled his mom's rusty Toyota behind a shiny black truck.

The gravel crunched beneath our feet as we walked up her long driveway. I heard bad pop music coming from the house. Shadows came alive on the screened-in balcony that rose over her carport.

By the time we got to the front door, I was sweating. I knocked, but no one answered. This trip already felt like a bad idea. Paul tried the door—it was unlocked. We shrugged and let ourselves in.

The upstairs was crammed with bodies, and their idiot voices magnified the mindless ringing in my ears. We maneuvered through the partiers. I recognized some of the kids. Not a single one recognized me.

The living room was hazy. I couldn't see Ali anywhere. Paul pushed ahead of me. He nodded toward the door of the balcony.

Ali was out there, standing beside a keg with her girlfriends. She didn't notice me until I slipped my hand around her waist. She jumped, startled, and then turned around and laughed drunkenly. She wrapped her arms around my neck, forgetting that a cigarette was dangling from her fingers. I started to cough. I swatted the air.

Ali apologized. She laughed again, softer this time. She didn't put the cigarette out.

Her girlfriends stared at me blankly for a moment, then started back into their conversation. The balcony was packed with people—if they weren't smoking cigarettes, they were smoking pot. If they weren't smoking pot, they were smoking *something*. I didn't understand how so much smoke could be trapped on a fucking outdoor patio.

I had to get away from it. Ali told me she would meet me in the living room. I pushed my way back through the crowd, leaving Paul standing alone, awkwardly trying to make eyes at a chick.

I sat down against the wall. Other kids stumbled around, spilling piss beer from plastic cups onto Ali's carpet. I saw a kid from my Spanish class, one of the ones who wrote the GET WELL cards. He didn't say hi. I don't think he'd ever known who I was.

I sat there alone. A girl bumped me, laughed. Beer covered my shoes.

Outside, I could hear Ali laughing. I wanted to disappear.

I sat there for ten more minutes. Paul finally abandoned his quest to find a girl who was special or slutty or drunk enough to give him the time of day. He sat with me inside.

Ali was still on the patio, laughing and talking. I could see her through the swaying crowd, smoking a joint with the girls in the same corner.

"Let's bail," I said.

"You wanna say later to Ali?"

"What's the point?"

Paul nodded. He helped me out of my chair. He held on to my arm as he pushed through the crowd.

In and out of their lives, and they don't even notice.

*   *   *

On Saturday, Nat told me that a band was doing a matinee show at the Y. He asked if I wanted to go. I was feeling pretty sorry for myself over the way things had gone at Ali's party and didn't want to get out of bed.

But Nat talked shit until I finally agreed to get dressed.

We picked up Paul and headed downtown. We pulled into the parking lot, but I was nervous to get out of the van.

When the kids outside saw our van, they reacted in the complete opposite way I expected. These punks and losers—most too shy to even talk to themselves—came to me as I stepped out of the car.

They hugged me. They told me they missed me. Many of them were kids I'd never spoken with and I knew that a few of them *hated* my band. But none of it mattered that afternoon—because I was one of their own.

When I saw Brody, he immediately brought up the auditions—when were we going to find a drummer? He had a few people in mind, he said again. I said that I was going back into the hospital Monday, so we'd have to wait until I got home.

He rolled his eyes.

The squeal of amplifiers came from inside the Y. We stopped our conversation and moved inside to see the show.

The band was already onstage. The guitarists were staring down at their tuners. The drummer looked bored. Nat suggested we stand in the back of the room.

"If a mosh pit breaks out," he said, "you probably don't want to be near it. Just a thought."

We moved to the back wall.

It was all for the best, anyway. Maybe I was imagining it, but I was starting to feel like no one *wanted* me up front, like no one wanted to be near me.

Everyone had been acting so nice—almost *too* nice— as soon as I showed up. But now I could feel them easing away. The show was starting. This was their time to have fun. They didn't want to think about cancer. No one needed this buzzkill.

I didn't feel sorry for myself this time, I just felt disappointed. In another life, I would've *never* stood in the back at a show. I would have wanted to yell. I would have wanted to mosh. But here I was, in the back, coldly observing a world that I suddenly felt half in, half out of.

The tinnitus made the fucking music unintelligible. It

was just one overpowering rumble, an earthquake inside of my head.

I looked at the crowd. I looked at their black T-shirts and skeleton patches and sighed. They raised their fists and middle fingers toward the stage.

Then, they chanted a eulogy.

TWELVE

Staggered Rays of Color and Light

1

There was no drama this time. There was no rushing, no doors busting open. We just parked in the two-dollar lot and strolled sleepily inside the hospital.

An off-duty cop monitored the elevators leading to the long-term care wards—he took one look at me, smiled sadly, and said, "Six."

When I arrived on the ward, they checked my blood pressure, temperature, height, weight—standard shit. Even though I'd been eating, I'd lost six more pounds.

A nurse walked us to my room. It was different, but the same.

This one was a softer blue. The nurse brought a hospital gown, neatly folded with a set of matching slippers on top of it. I went into the bathroom to change—there was no point bitching about it.

I stripped down to my underwear and tied the gown in a crooked shoestring knot. When I got out of the bathroom, I sat on the bed. The nurse took my hand and started searching for a vein.

———

There was no chemotherapy that first day back. It was like a warm-up—the hospital processed me into their system while I spent the day getting every test and scan they could cram in.

I drank the CT contrast, and I didn't even gag. They took sample after sample of my blood, but I didn't wince once. The scans were old news now.

They saved the green machine for last. Mom sat in the corner of the room reading a cheap thriller as the tech helped me onto the platform. I heard the machine start rumbling, then the platform moved slowly and it swallowed me whole.

When the scan was finally over, I dropped my feet back onto the cold tile. I was dazed. My brain was still shaking with the sound of the machine.

As Mom helped me out the door, I glanced at the techs going over the results on three separate computer monitors. I saw an outline of *my* body—filled with shapes and colors that reminded me of a news flash, a radar image of a storm. There were tiny little hurricanes moving inside me.

2

Day two.

Mid-afternoon the nurse brought the bags of poison. They dripped into the tube, into the needle, into the vein.

I knew what to expect from the treatment now. Mom closed the blinds and dimmed the lights. I unplugged the phone from the wall. I demanded *zero* stimulation, *zero* distractions—I needed to focus on not focusing. I needed to ignore all sensations. I needed to separate myself from consciousness like a skinny pale Buddha, trying not to puke and be sick and sad and miserable.

The poison hit my bloodstream.

I never lasted long.

*   *   *

In the hours before my injections—*if* I felt strong enough—I went on walks with Mom around the hospital. We made laps around the first-floor hallway. I moved ridiculously slowly, rolling my IV and using it for balance.

The walls of the hall displayed paintings done by other, younger patients—finger-turkeys and portraits of dogs, shit like that. We tried to pick our favorites.

There was a huge, open corridor that separated the two buildings of the hospital. Some rich person had donated a fish tank. The fish were bright exotic yellows and blues, oblivious to where they actually were. Watching them swim made me nauseous.

Across from the fish tank was the hospital chapel.

I didn't feel religious enough to walk in without seeming like a fraud. But when the doors of the chapel were open, I always looked inside. It was a small room with small pews that faced a large, crescent-shaped stained-glass window.

The window struck me. It depicted the image of a girl, wearing a plain white gown.

The *girl* fucking struck me. She held her heart up—toward the sky. Staggered rays of color and light shined down on her. Two hands reached out from the heavens toward her, this girl in crooked pieces below.

But she was always smiling.

Down the hall from the chapel was the hospice. I didn't notice it until the second time we passed. The entrance door was left open. I glanced inside. I saw a boy, about twelve, sitting in a wheelchair. His face was turned away from me. His hair was black. He was alone. A leg was missing.

I never looked at that door again.

3

Stacey found a bed for my mom at the Ronald McDonald House, right across the street. The parents of sick kids could stay there for free—it wasn't the nicest spot, but it was closer than any hotel. I could see it from my window.

I insisted she stay there. She didn't need to keep sleeping in a chair or on the small ledge beneath the sill of the window. She deserved a rest—or at least a fucking bed.

So Mom stayed with me every second of every day. She sat with me through the mornings, and through the brutal hours of my treatment. She stayed with me until the sun was down and the shifts had changed and the hallways of the ward were silent. Then, exhausted, she would kiss me on the head and go across the street.

In the nighttime, I was alone.

And when I was alone, I was *really* alone.

It's amazing how much having someone with me— just sitting in a chair reading, or watching the morning news—could normalize my situation. With no one to sit with or talk to, I had no way to guide where my mind went. . . .

The drugs helped my lonely thoughts, but only so much. My last round of pills came at nine in the evening, a few hours after the chemo effects began fading. As much as I hated the drugs, some nights I preferred feeling sick or stoned to facing the moments of total clarity that only came in those late hours.

Sometimes at night I plugged the cord back into the phone. I called home and said hi to Dad. I talked to Nat—*always* about the band. He told me that Brody had booked nine gigs around their Warped Tour dates. They were playing in Richmond, Buffalo, and all kinds of places. If he mentioned the other drummers waiting to audition for my spot, he always kept it brief. It seemed like things were rolling without a hitch. Maybe I wasn't as crucial to the band as I'd thought.

The first night I called Ali, we got into an argument.

Junior prom was in a few days—things had been moving so fast that I'd totally fucking forgotten about it. Ali, however, had definitely *not* forgotten about the prom. She still wanted to go. She just wanted to hang out and dance with her friends, then hit the after-parties. And besides, she already had a dress.

For some reason, the thought of Ali going to the prom sent me into a rage.

It was pathetic—she wasn't going with a date, or anything. She just wanted to have fun. All her friends were going. All the *normal* kids were going.

Maybe that's what pissed me off.

"Go ahead—*go*," I finally said. "I don't want anyone putting their lives on hold because of me. Fuck it."

Ali sighed. "I wish *you* were here to take me. I wish harder than you even know. But I can't just sit in my house all day, every day, all the time. It's driving me *crazy*."

"*WELL I FEEL SO SORRY FOR YOU!*"

The line went dead.

Shit. Dammit. Fucking idiot.

The hesitant talk. The constant stress—I saw a conflict growing inside Ali, the same way I saw it grow in my brother. Every time they got a chance to do something—go on tour, go to a stupid dance—they hesitated. It was like they were afraid to be normal anymore, because they knew that I couldn't.

The guilt of my existence was weighing down their lives. But I didn't want to hold them—or *anyone*—back. I wanted them to do the things I wasn't able to. I wanted them to do *everything*. I wanted them to live.

But that doesn't mean it didn't frustrate the hell out of me.

More and more, I felt myself becoming a resentful prick. The loneliness and sickness were no excuse. I always took my bad luck out on them. I always pushed those two the hardest. . . .

And where did it get me? Sitting in a room with a phone in my hand, listening to a dial tone.

Sitting in a room, alone.

*   *   *

Two nights later, when I was trying to sleep, I rolled over and ripped the IV from my arm. I jumped out of bed and flicked on the bathroom light to see what I'd done, and the reflection back was straight out of a horror movie.

The fluorescent lights made my face look translucent, but what really drove the image home was the blood squirting out of my arm and soaking my hospital gown. I pressed the call button and held my arm over the sink. Blood was everywhere. I thought I was going to faint. I didn't. I just stared at the ghost in the mirror and watched the blood spiral down.

4

On Saturday, as the nurse was hooking up my chemo, Mom said that Nat called to let her know he was driving up to visit. I said I wasn't in the mood to see anyone.

"Your brother is driving all the way up to see you. If you want to turn him away, you can do it yourself."

I didn't answer her. The nurse had started the drip. I felt the sensation spread through my throat and gut.

Concentrate NOW—nothing, nothing, nothing.

*   *   *

It was eight thirty at night. Mom was already gone. When I heard the knock I was in bed reading, waiting on my last dose of pills.

"Yeah?"

The door opened. Ali stood there alone. I put my book down and stared at her. She didn't have on a prom dress—only ripped shorts, and my Bad Religion T-shirt.

"Whoa. What are you doing *here*?"

Ali shrugged and smiled. She walked toward my bed.

Why hadn't I wanted her to go to prom? Why did I have to scream and bitch and guilt her to the point that she ended up here, wasting her night in this horrible place just wasting away with me?

I wanted to tell her that she'd made a mistake. I wanted to tell her that she should have gone with her friends. She shouldn't be in some cramped, puke-smelling hospital room with this jaded prick. . . .

But all that I said was—"Where's Nat?"

"In the hall. He said he'd give us some time alone."

I cleared my throat.

"Well, you still wanna dance?" I asked. My words came out hoarse.

Ali laughed. "In here?"

"Why not? Help me up."

I pushed my feet down onto the floor. Ali held my shoulders until I steadied myself. I put my hands loosely on her waist.

She ran her hands over my shoulders and back behind my neck. She moved closer. When she pressed against me, my hospital gown draped over the curves of her body. . . . She eased her head onto my shoulder.

We swayed—*slow*.

Back. Forth. Back. Forth. *Slow*—like branches moving together in a breeze.

I breathed in the smell of her hair. I memorized her heat.

"What about music?" she said softly. "Don't we need some music?"

"I can hear it if you can," I said.

And I could.

THIRTEEN

A/S/L

1

Life at home picked up speed. Everyone seemed so damn busy.

Nat was rehearsing alone in the basement. Finals were approaching, and that was something even my friends took semi-seriously. Dad was working crazy long hours.

He and Mom were stressed about money. They didn't say anything, but I knew. One morning, I found them going over my medical bills at the dinner table. I was on Mom's insurance plan, the one she got through work—aka the job she hadn't gone to since she started taking care of me.

But that same evening, she told me she was thinking of going back to the office until my next round of treatments. I said that it was fine.

So now, I spent most of my day alone. Before Mom went to the office in the morning, she put my medications out and left a fresh trash can at my bedroom door in case I got nauseous.

I spent most of my time sleeping or watching daytime TV. The "A Transvestite Hooker Got Me Pregnant"–type shit. I think it was comforting to see people whose lives were even more fucked than mine.

I spent more time online than I used to, assuming our modem would connect. America Online was an amazing thing—there was *nothing* like it. I could look up band sites, I could look up porn—the Internet kicked total ass.

AOL also allowed me to meet new people, or kinda meet them, at least. There were chat rooms—*thousands* of them—where I could talk to perfect strangers about anything I wanted. Day by day, I started snooping through them.

There were punk rock chats and skateboard chats. There were *tons* of sex chats, pretty much any kind I coulda dreamed up, but the people in them were a little weird. Okay, a lot weird. There were chats about anything and everything.

One day, I found a chat room called CancerKidz. I moved my arrow over the tab, hesitating for just a moment before I clicked it. The chat opened. There was only one other user inside. It was a girl.

Nocomply11: Hey, what's up?

CynamnGirl84: hi A/S/L?

Nocomply11: 17/M/WV U?

CynamnGirl84: 16/F/IL

Sixteen? The number filled me with twisted excitement. There wasn't anyone on the cancer ward my age. It was beginning to feel like I was the first person in history to get cancer who wasn't either a little kid or a geriatric. The prospect of finding a teenage cancer patient to talk to—even one I couldn't see—was something that I'd pretty much given up on.

My new 16/F friend's real name was Babs. Babs, from the suburbs of Chicago. Babs, in the fucking cancer chat room.

I was online for the next three hours, chatting with her about normal stuff . . . music, the city, whatever. It took a while for me to ask why she was in CancerKidz.

Babs told me she didn't have cancer. It was her friend who was sick. They'd been chatting together right before I entered the room.

Part of me was let down, as messed up as that sounds. She asked why *I* was in the chat room. My fingers moved before I realized I was typing. I told her the whole story—I may have exaggerated how famous my band was, but the rest of the story was true.

I didn't know how bad I'd needed to talk about cancer to someone who wasn't a friend, brother, girlfriend, or parent. I couldn't speak openly with those close to me— because the words hurt. So I typed it all out to this girl, fifteen paragraphs of rants, frustrations, and fears. . . .

Before she could respond, my Internet cut out.
Shit.

It took me fifteen minutes to get the modem to reconnect. The chat room was empty. *Double shit.* My 16/F/IL was gone.

I leaned on the desk, frustrated. I wondered if I'd ever speak to her again. I decided to wait it out for a while.

I left the chat window open and surfed over to my favorite website—HTown Punx. It wasn't really a website, more like a message board. This kid Kris made it to help let people know what shows were coming up around town—Paul, and every other promoter, posted show info and band websites.

But anyone could post on HTown Punx. Kids wrote show reviews, band suggestions, lineup changes, rumors, and anything semi-interesting going down in Huntington.

I wanted to see if Brody had posted anything about a fill-in drummer.

I scrolled down the message thread until I saw our band name. *This is dated three weeks ago,* I thought. *He sure didn't waste any time.*

I clicked it. The post opened—wait, what?

Posted by: FUCKU-182

Defiance of Authority is such fucking lame fake punk. They fucking SHOULD be called DOA because they have a drummer who is going to fucking die of cancer before they even get the chance to sell out, and I hope he does. I hope his fucking brother drives their van off a cliff and kills every poser fuck inside it.

I reread the post, confused. Who would ever say this crazy shit? Why would anyone say they hoped I *died*?

My mind drew a blank.

I didn't recognize the user name. I went back to the main thread and continued to scroll down.

Since I was diagnosed with cancer, FUCKU-182 had

posted about our band three times. Each post was worse than the last. Surprisingly, I wasn't really hurt. Only pissed. The words turned red in my mind.

I was so mad I was shaking. My fingers made the keyboard keys chatter like teeth. I read the posts over and over. I committed them to memory. I looked for clues. I was going to find out who wrote these words and then shove every single syllable back down their fucking throat.

2

It took three days to unmask the anonymous poster.

My friend Angela—an older chick who basically *lived* on that message board—had started asking around for me. I logged on one day to find her e-mail waiting.

> I'm pretty sure FUCKU-182 is Frank Parker. He goes to school with you guys, right? Hope you are feeling better, I miss you!

Frank Parker—nope, I still didn't recognize the name.

I looked through my closet, until I found last year's HHS yearbook. I scanned our entire class—no luck. I flipped up to the class ahead of us—nothing. I flipped to the grade below mine—*pay dirt*.

A photo of a chubby, hook-nosed kid peered at me. His mouth was half open, in what I assumed was a smile. His black hair hung over his zit-marked face. I recognized this kid—*barely*.

We'd never talked. I'd never hung out with him. He was a stranger.

I wasn't sure what to think. Why would a stranger say that stuff? Why would *anyone* say that kind of stuff?

More important—*what was I going to do about it?*

Normally the answer would be nothing, of course. I was never one to stick up for myself, even under the worst circumstances. I'd get beat up, shamed, and humiliated before I would ever take a stand.

But for some reason, this felt different. I don't know, maybe I'd simply had enough. The cancer, the band, my hair, my *life*—and now *this*?

I couldn't get over it. I just couldn't fucking let it go.

3

I kept my plan simple.

First, I would find out Frank Parker's class schedule. I'd drive to the school and wait outside his second-period class (for maximum hallway traffic). When Frank came out of class, he'd see *me*—standing right in front of him.

Before he could collect himself, I would calmly yell, *"Who's DOA now, motherfucker!,"* spit on him, punch him in the face (breaking his nose and knocking him unconscious), and then disappear into a cheering crowd of onlookers.

It seemed pretty cut-and-dried.

I knew that I shouldn't tell Nat about *any of it.*

He would never let me get into a fight. Nat would want to deal with Frank himself, and that didn't seem fair to me. *I* wanted to be the one. Frank needed to see my hairless, shrunken face before I knocked him on his ass.

So I enlisted Paul. He came with all the loyalty of a brother, but only half of the guilty conscience. And he was totally into my plan.

Because of his gig on yearbook staff, Paul could roam the school as much as he wanted, come and go as he pleased. He'd be able to do recon on Frank, pick me up, cheer me on, and drop me back at my house before Nat even knew what had happened.

The plan was fucking foolproof.

* * *

"Who's DOA now, motherfucker!" I shouted at my bathroom mirror.

I scowled. I cleared my throat.

"Who's DOA *now*, mother*fucker!*"

I'd spent the morning hyping myself up. I skipped my first dose of medication—I didn't want the pills to make me groggy. I could take them when I got home. This beatdown wouldn't take long.

I wasn't wearing a hat or a sweatshirt—I wanted Frank to *see* me. I wanted him to have visions of me while he lay unconscious and bleeding on the floor.

A car horn sounded from outside.

Beep, be-be, beep-beep, beep beep—Paul.

I hurried out the door. I kept running my lines. . . .

We were pushing it on time.

Frank had Algebra second period. Room 237. Class ended at nine fifty-five. But by the time we got to the school and parked, it was already nine forty-seven.

Paul rushed into the building. I did my best to keep up. I had to stop and catch my breath before we made it to the stairwell.

Nine fifty-three—we were on the second floor. I was panting. I willed my legs not to buckle. I looked from left to right—Room 228, Room 233 . . .

"Dude!" Paul hissed.

He pointed. I looked—*237*. Bingo.

I collapsed against the wall.

"Time?" I wheezed.

Paul checked his watch. We had thirty seconds to go.

I clenched my left fist. I stared at the door of 237. I caught my breath.

A surge of adrenaline hit me. My exhaustion became nothing but background noise. Something inside called my messed-up body to *action*!

The fucking bell rang. I didn't fucking flinch.

I moved toward the door. I felt like a boxer entering his first round.

Kids walked out. A girl with a pink backpack nearly ran into me. Another moved past me to get to her locker. I didn't fucking flinch. I clenched my fucking fist *tighter*.

I didn't see Frank Parker anywhere.

I waited. *Nothing*.

I backed up a little, fading into the hallway's growing crowd.

Then, all of a sudden, there he was.

Frank fucking Parker.

He was taller than I expected. His eyes were too close to his nose. His hair was as black and messy as an oil slick.

He didn't look at me. He didn't look at *anyone*. He kept his eyes fastened downward, the same way I used to do.

I took a deep breath.

"Hey!" I yelled.

Frank Parker fucking *stopped*.

Those beady eyes met mine. If he recognized me, it didn't show.

"Who's DOA," I began. But I froze. I couldn't remember my fucking line! The chemo brain hit me at the worst possible time!

I winged it—it came out as "Uhhh . . . um . . ."

Screw the speech, I decided.

I spit on him. I was too far away for my spit to actually make it to his face. It landed on his shoulder—at least I'm pretty sure it did.

Screw the spitting.

I tensed my arm and swung my fist. Flesh crashed into flesh.

Frank didn't fucking move.

I hit him right on the cheek. I hit him with everything I had. *He didn't move.* I'd put my whole being into that punch.

But my fist just kind of *stuck* to his cheek—it was still fucking there! I was leaning on his face. I was using him like some kind of crutch.

I breathed hard through my mouth. My vision was cloudy. I didn't know what to do.

Paul stood watching—he didn't know what to do. We didn't have a contingency plan—not for *this*.

Frank stepped back. He swatted my hand away like an inconvenience.

The swat was all it took. I went down.

I wasn't sure what was happening. People were moving and the hall was moving and everything was going wrong. I was sprawled in the middle of the floor. I couldn't catch my breath. I tried to get up, but I didn't have the strength.

My body lay there, useless.

Through the corner of my glasses, I saw Paul jump on Frank. He was swinging wildly, as he always did when he fought. A teacher rushed onto the scene, and Paul accidentally punched her.

Feet smashed around my head as the onlookers moved closer. I looked at the ceiling. I focused on the cheap foam panels and tried to control my breath. I closed my eyes and let the air flow into my nose and out my lips, into my nose and out my lips.

A sneaker smack exploded beside my ear.

Into my nose and out my lips.

I waited to hear something snap.

FOURTEEN

Cheap Thrills

1

I was low, man.

My "fight" at school was a disaster. Paul was suspended for the rest of the year. So was Frank.

Nat was pissed at me. Nat was pissed at Paul. Nat was *pissed* that Frank got suspended—he was AWOL. Retaliation was now impossible.

I was too embarrassed to speak to anyone. I didn't even get online. I didn't feel like I was worth anyone's time. *Pathetic* x *a billion* = *me.*

Worse, every day that passed was a day closer to summer. Brody asked me to make a list of songs that I wanted drummers to audition with. He said he'd found the perfect drummer.

Pathetic x *a trillion* = *my fucking ass.*

I felt about as worthless as a dude could feel.

*   *   *

I was lying on the floor of the empty living room, watching TV.

209

Jenny Jones wore one of her pink skirt-suits. She was asking her audience if they thought the girl onstage should leave her husband for his brother, or the brother for the husband—I couldn't tell how the crowd was leaning.

I switched the TV off.

Why was I wasting my day like this? Why wasn't I playing drums?

How are you going to play drums again if you can't breathe? If you don't get stronger? If you don't get in better shape? Shit, you're forty pounds lighter—chemo did the hard part. Now all you have to do is push your body a little. . . .

Exercise—come on, I was too weak to get off the couch most days. I'd never been athletic, or anywhere close to physically fit. I wouldn't even know where to begin.

I was too weak to do much. Running and jogging were out, obviously. I wondered if I should check with Dr. Ranalli before I did anything stupid.

But a voice inside kept giving me shit.

You've got nothing to lose by trying now—*you're tapped, dude. You've got nothing.*

As soon as that thought entered my mind, I rolled onto my chest and pushed. There was no thought, no planning.

I just pushed.

I couldn't believe how hard it was to do a push-up. My arms wobbled. My fingers dug into the carpet and I pushed myself up until my elbows were nearly straight.

I counted it—*one.*

I dropped back down quickly, trying to use the momentum to propel my body back into the air.

It worked—*two.*

I tried another. I only made it about halfway up before my arms buckled under me. I fell facedown on the carpet.

I grinned—*two and a half.*

*   *   *

The next day, I did a total of *six* push-ups.

I could only manage a few at a time, so I spread them out through my day. I probably could've done more than six, but I puked after lunch—vomiting takes more energy than you'd think.

On the third day, I did *twenty*. Twenty!

Twenty fucking push-ups in a single day—I was elated. Before my diagnosis, I never woulda been able to do twenty push-ups, not even in the start/stop method I adopted. So I don't know how I was able to do it now, while on chemo. I think I was running on willpower alone.

Exercising didn't make me tired—no more tired than I already was, at least. It made me feel *excited*. It made me feel like I still had a say in *something*.

I went into my parents' bedroom. I opened the closet. I dug through a pile of Mom's shoes until I found them— her five-pound aerobic dumbbells.

I picked them up.

They didn't feel very heavy. I curled my arms up a few times. The weights felt heavier. I curled a few more. My arms turned to butter.

I dropped the weights. I shook out my arms. I caught my breath. I stared at the weights. . . .

I picked them up again.
I arched my back.
I pulled.

* * *

The next morning, my entire body ached and the port in my arm fucking *throbbed*. My muscles were tense. It was an awesome feeling—I couldn't believe there were muscles beneath this pale, droopy skin.

I rolled out of bed. I put on my glasses, groaned, stretched, pissed, and walked out into the foyer. Our house seemed so empty.

I knocked on my parents' door—no answer.

I went back into their closet. I pulled out the weights. *I shouldn't be able to do this,* I thought to myself.

And then I did it.

2

That year of my life was defined by extremes.

My band was playing in an empty basement . . . my band was in *Rolling Stone*.

I was a cheeseburger away from obesity . . . I was emaciated beyond recognition.

I couldn't get a date . . . I was banging a cheerleader.

I didn't do drugs . . . I took handfuls of pills and mainlined poison.

There was no in-between. Not for me.

And those two weeks were no different—the fight with Frank had made me face the fact that I was broken, that my body had been ravaged by the war within it. That truth had pushed me lower than I'd even thought possible. The more I rallied against my negative thoughts, the faster I sank.

And you know what? The sinking feeling came with a strange kind of peace.

All the uncertainty I felt was gone, replaced with the knowledge that I had nowhere to go but *up*. I could try to get my head above water. *Or* I could stay where I was, and drift wherever I may. This was *my* call. It was the first time since my diagnosis that I felt like a choice was up to me.

So I regained a small amount of control over my own fate. I was imposing *my* will—and it was working. It opened my heart to possibilities. I started thinking, *If I can do* this, *then I can do* that. *And this. And that . . .*

I heard subliminal messages in my old records—all the rebel anthems in the world were now united against a common enemy. Sure, I knew that the songs had nothing to do with my situation . . . but their fuck-you attitude did. The attitude was contagious.

When I didn't have the will to get out of bed, or the strength to push myself off the floor, I would try to think like a punk rocker—one who needs no other reason to act besides the cheap thrill of defiance.

School was almost over now. Soon, the summer would begin. I didn't care anymore.

Nothing would change for me. I would stay focused. The more alone I got, the more I could *focus*. I didn't need visitors. I didn't need bullshit.

The time came for me to return to the hospital. I welcomed it.

The sooner I could finish that round of chemo, the sooner I could deal with cancer on my own fucking terms.

3

Hospital. Cancer ward.

After the results of my first-day tests, Dr. Ranalli decided we should change the drugs in my "chemo cocktail." The bleomycin was causing side effects far beyond puking and shitting—my tinnitus and nerve damage continued to get worse.

More important, the drug was causing the muscles of my heart, lungs, and kidneys to harden, making them work less effectively. Dr. Ranalli feared that another dose would cause further damage.

The drug he switched with the bleomycin was similar, but less toxic. He warned that I might get a little more nauseous, but said that the long-term side effects would be minimal.

I didn't care. I was willing to take whatever he told me to take. Fuck risks. Fuck aftereffects.

I'd worry about aftereffects *after*. I was thinking in the now.

*　*　*

Dr. Ranalli came back to my room during the second day of chemo, after a discussion with the specialists in Indiana.

The tumor was shrinking considerably. Dr. Einhorn's

team was still confident that with surgery, and a few more rounds of chemotherapy, I had a chance at beating this thing.

Dr. Ranalli was trying to organize a meeting between Dr. Einhorn and me. He said that after one more round of chemotherapy, they would be prepared to operate. They wanted to examine me in person before the surgery was scheduled.

So, after the next round of chemo, we would be driving to Indiana. After that, I was going to take a break from treatment—before *and* after the operation—so my body wasn't completely depleted.

Only a couple more rounds of treatment would follow.

Then I would be totally done. I might even get to start my senior year with everyone else.

Surgery. A few more sick weeks. Then everything gets back to normal.

No problem.

FIFTEEN

Pity Tucks

1

The landscape rose up in soft green arches, and the black-topped street that ran straight through town looked like a river of tar. The humidity and the smell of catfish overwhelmed the senses. Even the trees slouched over in exhaustion.

Another West Virginia summer began.

To me, the summer meant company.

The school year ended with an uneventful shrug. My parents didn't even ask to see our grades. None of us cared.

Nat was home now. Paul came over every day. As tour loomed closer, the house would become more and more alive. The time had come to audition drummers.

I was trying not to act jaded about it. I mean, finding a fill-in had been my idea to begin with—but that didn't make it any easier. I kept reminding myself that things were how they were—I could either deal with them or give up.

Like I said, there were no more in-betweens.

The first drummer who auditioned was Brody's boy, Doyle. He played drums in some emo band from Ashland.

He arrived at our house in a small blue hatchback. The windows were covered with mud. I couldn't see the driver.

I waited on the porch, probably as nervous as he was. Doyle ducked out of the front seat—he was at least six and a half feet tall. His hair was spiked into thick, uneven clumps that made him even taller. He had a perfectly round beer gut. He wore all black and a studded leather belt with a skull on the buckle.

A pair of chipped drumsticks stuck out of his right pocket.

Doyle walked onto the porch. He came straight to *me*. He shook my hand.

"It's sure as hell nice to meet ya," he said. "Wanted to tell ya how much it means to get a chance to play with y'all."

His accent was so thick I had to strain to understand him.

"We're just glad you could do it!" Brody said loudly.

Doyle didn't notice.

"Really, man, you're one of the best drummers 'round here. I ain't gonna fuck up all them parts you wrote."

"You'll be *great*!" Brody said, walking between us. "Let's get to it, big man."

He slapped Doyle on the back. Doyle shrugged. We walked single file down into the basement.

* * *

I wanted to hate him. I really did.

But Doyle was a *fan* of the band. Doyle saw me as a musician, not a fucking cancer patient. He treated me like a peer, not a living corpse.

Plus, I had to admit—Doyle was a damn good drummer.

He looked ridiculous towering over my kit. But he'd learned every single song on the audition list. He played simplified versions of the parts, removing the fills, keeping it straight. It was strange to watch my band play without me. But Doyle laid down a solid foundation for Nat and Brody to do their thing.

They jammed for a half hour. When they finished "Without You," Doyle sat on my drum throne and looked at me, trying to gauge what I thought.

The roundness of his stomach extended to his knees. He kept staring at me. He looked like a puppy, begging to be adopted.

I stared back at him, expressionless.

Then, slowly, I gave him the thumbs-up.

What else *could* I do? Tour was coming. We had to find someone. If it wasn't Doyle, it would be someone else— or, shit, what if no one else was good enough? By the time I was cured, we would have already blown it. This funny hillbilly was my best chance to keep the dream alive.

I felt like it was the right decision. And a *temporary* decision. Doyle was just a fill-in. All of this shit was just temporary.

As the three of them set up a practice schedule I excused myself. I needed to lie down.

2

Rehearsals ran from noon until five, four days a week. I sat in the basement for the first few, giving Doyle notes and helping with ideas for the set. But after a while, I left them alone. They were sounding tighter as a separate unit—I didn't want to interfere with that.

I stayed upstairs, exercising out of sight.

That last round of chemo was a blow to my workouts, and getting back into the swing of it was tough. I was exhausted. I was frustrated. But I kept trying. If I paced myself, I knew I could do it.

Ali spent a lot of time at the pool that summer. She lay in the grass with her friends, smoking cigarettes and pounding vodka from empty Sprite bottles. She invited me to come with her a few times, but I was still supposed to stay out of the sun.

One day, Ali showed up at my house with a blue plastic kiddie pool that had been sitting out in front of Love Hardware. She saw it on the way to work, and she bought it on sale.

I filled the pool up with the garden hose. Ali changed inside. I positioned the pool at the bottom of the back stairs—now she could sit in the sun, and I could stay under the stoop's tin awning. I grabbed a small trash can, in case I felt sick.

If Ali and I were together that summer, chances were she was in her pool. The water couldn't have been more than twelve inches deep; the pool was barely big enough for even such a small girl.

She liked to wear this purple bikini (*Jesus*). I can still see her, leaning back on the edge of the pool, her stomach and top glistening as she stretched. Her freckles practically *glowed*.

She would float in that water and talk with me for hours. We spent entire afternoons that way—me in the shade, her out there in the sunlight. She rose from the deep, my lost queen of Atlantis. She didn't belong in a world like mine.

I sat in the shadows, squinting into the light.

3

Having a birthday really pissed me off.

I mean, what the fuck? I was about to go back to the hospital for chemo session number four. Now, suddenly, I was supposed to be stoked about turning eighteen? My life was *supposed* to be on *hold*.

Everyone knew it. It was hard enough for me to watch my twin brother progress—continuing on and on and on. I didn't want a party to celebrate a transition that everyone damn well knew I wasn't making.

But Mom insisted on doing *something*—so she ordered pizzas and picked up a Baskin-Robbins ice cream cake. I invited as few people over as possible.

Ali, Paul, Doyle, Tyson, Ashley, Angela, Brody, and Jamie all stopped by at some point in the day. Our grandparents came by. Random relatives came by.

Paul gave me a hardback copy of *The Count of Monte Cristo*, one of my favorite books. I got Nat a new skate deck for the road. Nat got me a Black Flag jacket, a new beanie, and a new hair dryer.

"Something to look forward to," he joked.

Ali handed me her gift last. It was wrapped in pink notebook paper. I tore it open.

It was a framed photograph—a picture of the two of us. The picture David snapped on the day they found the deathmass rotting my chest . . .

The amateur black-and-white processing made the photo look out of another time, one where cancer and pain had no place. This was just a boy and a girl. Smiling. Careless. Healthy. Untouched.

I realized that my hand was shaking. I sat the picture down.

"Do you like it?" Ali asked.

She was smiling her smile.

I cleared my throat. "I love it, baby."

I smiled back at her. I wondered if the kids in the photo would even recognize my face.

*   *   *

By eight o'clock, the party finally died. Ali was working the night shift at the drive-thru. The other relatives and friends drifted off on their own.

Mom was finishing off a bottle of wine. Dad was watching TV. Paul sat around the kitchen table with Nat and me, counting our birthday cash.

My relatives were extra generous that year.

Nat decided that it was the perfect time to tell our parents he'd be using this cash to get tattoos.

Mom told him he couldn't.

She demanded that he didn't.

She *commanded* him—he *would not.*

They argued and argued about it. There was nothing she could actually do—he was eighteen now. It was his money. But it was her maternal duty to fucking freak out.

So the birthday party I never wanted ended in a screaming match. Nat finally grabbed the keys to the van and bailed. He didn't say where he was going.

Mom downed the rest of her wine and went upstairs.

"Jesus," Paul said, once she was gone. "When your ma gets white-wine drunk, *look out.*"

Dad walked into the kitchen.

"All right," he said, clapping his hands, "we ready?"

"For what?"

Dad looked around. "Where's your brother?"

"Uh, didn't you hear him and Mom going at it?"

Dad shook his head.

"So Nat left?"

"Yep."

"Ah well, his loss." He looked at Paul. "I guess this one is going to have to take your brother's place tonight."

"Take his place doing what?" Paul asked.

"Celebrating."

* * *

Dad did taxes for lots of businesses around Huntington. One of his more lucrative clients was the owner of Southern X-Posure, the only strip club near town. It was outside the city limits, in a renovated Ponderosa

Steakhouse off the highway between Barboursville and Milton.

I couldn't believe we were actually here. The parking lot of the club was packed. I heard the pulse of drum machines before we were even inside.

The door guy knew Dad's first name. He didn't charge us a cover. Paul wasn't even eighteen, but he didn't check IDs.

Dad handed me a wad of dollar bills.

"Happy birthday, big boy," he said.

We followed the music inside.

Truckers and college kids sat hovering over their drinks. The haze of neon and smoke made it hard to see anything except the stage. The walls were completely covered in mirrors.

Dad went to the bar as Paul and I stumbled around, not sure what to do. I watched the girl onstage, I think she was a redhead. Her boobs were spaced too far apart to be real. She spotted me and headed my way.

I was frozen in place.

She smiled and leaned down to me. All it took was her pressing her tits together and snapping her garter for me to hold out the entire wad of cash in my trembling hand.

She took it all.

She winked—*Thanks, kid.*

"Fucking Christ!" Dad yelled behind me.

He and Paul were at a table near the back. I walked over, embarrassed.

"You don't *ever* give a girl all your money!" he said.

Paul laughed.

"I mean—how much am I supposed to give them?"

Dad shrugged and took a drink.

"It depends, but shit, I wouldn't give that one more than a pity tuck. Maybe some spare change."

Paul, thinking he was serious, started pulling dimes and quarters from his front pocket. He made it halfway to the stage before Dad dragged him back to the table.

A stripper walked up and sat in my lap.

She was younger than the dancer onstage. Her hair was bleached, the way mine used to be. She had a diamond belly ring that bounced when she moved. Her heels were a hundred inches long.

The weight of her ass pushed down upon me. She spoke from over her shoulder.

"What's your name, baby?"

"Uh . . . Rob . . ."

"Hi, baby," she said. "I'm Contagious."

Dad laughed. Contagious didn't pay any mind.

She took the hat off my head and put it on. She rubbed my hairless scalp. She didn't mention the port hanging off my arm. It was too dark for her to see that I was just a ghost.

Contagious asked if I wanted a *private* dance.

Before I could answer, my dad said yes—I definitely wanted one. He pulled more cash out of his back pocket. He handed it to me. Contagious took my hand and helped me out of my chair.

She was patient with me. She held my hand. I focused on the ass of the woman who led me toward the back of the club.

We came to a dark hallway. Private booths ran down each side.

Contagious led me to the back of the hall. We passed dances in progress. I didn't make eye contact with the other men. The girls all kept their eyes closed.

Contagious sat me in a stain-covered chair without armrests. She rubbed my head again. Her eyes looked sad for the both of us.

She straddled my waist with her thick legs.

She wrapped her arms around my neck, the way Ali used to do. She leaned in like she wanted to kiss me, but then nuzzled her face in my neck. I felt hot breath on my skin. She leaned back.

Contagious undid her top. I tried to relax. She moved her stomach and tits against my face. They squashed over me like half-empty water balloons. I tried to breathe through the flesh. I smelled cocoa butter, and Wal-Mart perfume.

Above the booth was a single red bulb. It flickered and burnt through the smoke in the air like our own little tired sunset.

SIXTEEN

A Sense of an Ending

1

Nat and I sat in the basement. We talked ink.

We were all stoked about getting tattooed. We decided that our first one should be matching—one big piece that came together when we put our arms side by side, real "Wonder Twins—activate!"-type shit.

I wasn't allowed to get tattooed, though, not while I was still getting chemo. It was too much toxicity for my body to handle. Nat, however, was good to go.

He wanted to get his half of the tattoo before he left for tour. We spent tons of time trying to decide on a design. While the two of us discussed tattoos, it was hard for me to keep my eyes from drifting to the map Nat had posted on the basement wall.

It was the United States—torn from a gas station atlas. He had the highways and side routes of their summer tour traced in black—he'd used a felt-tip pen to mark each show city with a bright red star.

I stared at the black-lined highways—27, 35, 64, 77, 99, *138*, north, east, south, west—but it all seemed like one long road to me.

I ran my finger down and then left—Cleveland to Indianapolis.

I was going to Indy to meet Dr. Einhorn in less than two weeks. I ran my finger back up to Cleveland—the band was playing there, near the end of the tour. I tried to measure the distance.

My finger moved farther west, dipping through the curves of the road. I traced Highway 70 through Minnesota—toward Highway 40 through Oklahoma— into the Wild West.

I kept going.

Texas bled into the American deserts. I imagined tires crunching over rattlesnake eggs and Indian burial grounds. . . . I kept going.

That fucking road went straight to Hollywood Boulevard.

Nat's map made those places seem real. Every direction led somewhere, everywhere, anywhere but *here*.

White lines stretched endlessly through my mind. If you could make it onto that highway, you could make it outta Huntington. As long as my brother came back for me, I could make it out too.

2

Hospital. Cancer ward. Chemotherapy. Round four.

A strip of tape came loose on my hand. I studied it. The drugs moved slowly.

I groaned. I used my free hand to massage my temples. I shut my eyes in one long, pointless wince.

I held out for six more minutes. I felt the drugs bubble up in my guts. Six and a half . . .

I leaned over the side of my chair and began to vomit.

Chemo made me just as sick as it always had. That part would never get easier. But at least it was easier for me to *focus*.

I didn't whine anymore. I didn't complain.

There were no more surprises left. I was almost done—in a few days I would trade this hospital for the one in Indiana. Then I would be home. Then I would be *back*—this was the big one. They would cut this corpse of a tumor out of my fucking body forever.

It was almost July. Nat would be on the road soon, probably the same time I was having surgery. I didn't mind—he needed to go. They were *our* songs, and I was ready for people out in the real world to hear them.

By the time Nat was back home, I would be as good as new.

Better, even—I made a vow to exercise even more after the surgery. I wouldn't be so tired, so I could push myself until I had the strength to play drums again.

That was the goal, the only thing that mattered. I would practice more than ever before—theory, techniques, all the boring shit I used to skip over.

By the time Nat was home, the hair would be back on my head. I was going to dye it black, like his. I was going to get tattooed, like him.

I was going to carry my weight in the band. I was going to pick up the slack.

If I had a few more shots of chemo down the line, so what?

Because after I would be *CURED*.

Everything would get back on track. It would be better than fucking ever.

So while the treatments still wrecked my body, they took less of a toll on my heart. I didn't need to reflect anymore—I just wanted to get it done. Because for the first time in a long time, I had a sense of an ending.

I would get done. I would get out.

From Columbus to Indianapolis. From Indianapolis to home. Then straight back again. Then back again.

And from there . . . the world.

3

"You ever been to Chicago?" I asked the janitor.

"Can't say I have," he said.

"What about LA?"

"Nope."

He mopped the bathroom. I had visions of maps.

"I went all the way to Germany once, though," he said.

"Damn. Really?"

"Mm-hm, ol' Deutschland, back when I was in the service. Hell, I probably wasn't much older than you."

"Did you dig it?"

He shrugged. "I was stationed outside K-Town—pretty country, but boring. Peacetime and all."

"Bummer."

"Went to Hamburg once on leave, though."

"Was it cool?"

He grinned at me.

"You heard of the red-light district, Youngblood?"

"I think so," I said, propping myself up in bed.

He whistled.

"Is it like, strip joints?"

He shook his head. His grin went *wide*.

"They'll strip—but that ain't all. I'm talkin' blocks of nothing but tramps, girls standing in windows in nothing but G-strings."

"Jesus, really?"

"Well, the lights are more pink than red, now that I think on it. But the G-string part is true. You just walk right up and point—just like a doggie in a window."

"Whoa."

He laughed. "Those European women will *do things*, boy! I spent three months' pay in one damn night. I start sweating just thinking about it."

I thought of Ali. I thought of Contagious. My drugged-up mind swirled breasts and thighs and legs and endless bodies, mixing and matching every girl I'd ever seen into one sex-fueled mystery girl of the night, one sacred goddess waiting for me to get better. Waiting somewhere far away from here, out in the heart of the world.

*　　*　　*

On the day before the last day, the phone rang in my room. Mom answered—it was Nat. I waved it over to the bed.

"What's up?" I said weakly.

"Wanted to tell ya I'm going to House of Ink tomorrow night, to get our tattoo," he said.

"Already?" I asked. I had thought we would go together.

"Yeah, tomorrow is the only time they can fit me in before tour."

"Okay," I said.

"Dad is actually on a plane to Columbus right now, so he can ride with y'all to Indy. He told me he wouldn't mention it to Mom—so you don't either. Paul and Tyson are going down to the shop with me. Ali too, maybe."

*　*　*

"Can I get tattooed?" I asked.

Stacey and Dr. Ranalli were in my room, the way they always were before I was discharged. My question made them laugh. Dad and Mom were both there. It didn't make them laugh.

We had a long drive through Indiana ahead of us.

"I expected questions relating to your vacation from chemo, but that's a new one," Dr. Ranalli said.

"All the chemo will be outta my system, right? So am I allowed to get tattooed before I come back? Is it safe?"

"Say he isn't allowed," Mom said.

Dr. Ranalli cleared his throat.

"Let me put it this way—from a medical standpoint, getting tattooed should be safe. From any other standpoint, you're on your own."

4

Indiana is eighty-six percent corn. Seriously—just miles and miles of fucking corn. Fields of corn lined the highway, budding around us like some golden dream. The sunshine reflected off the cornstalks. The world was a beautiful glare.

The map was one thing. This was something else. I was farther west than I had ever been. The changes in the landscape rocked me. The tug of *freedom* pulled at my heart.

I passed out sometime before we neared the city. The chemo cocktail still sloshed through my bloodstream.

I awoke as Dad drove slowly through the campus of Indiana University, looking for the hospital. I saw a group of girls in short red shorts. I waved.

The hospital was on the next block. It was the biggest hospital I'd been to yet—not a small-town hospital, not a children's hospital—a *big-city hospital*. The ceiling of the atrium must have stretched twenty stories high.

The wheelchairs had long wicker backs. They looked like luxury rocking chairs. *When you admire the quality of wheelchairs,* I thought, *you know your priorities are fucked.*

We found the elevators—going up.

Dr. Einhorn's office was on the fifth floor. His waiting room was filled with nothing but Lance Armstrong stuff—books, bracelets, pamphlets, photos—my parents seemed impressed.

We waited a half hour. I started feeling sick. I walked off to find a bathroom to puke in.

The walk turned into a panicked run.

I found a men's room just in time. I was through the door like gangbusters, and I rushed blindly into the first metallic stall, lurched forward, and let go. If there was someone inside it, I could apologize later.

I don't know how long I was in there.

When I eventually heard Dad calling for me, I didn't even realize I'd fallen asleep in the stall.

*   *   *

Dad rousted me up and led me to the exam room. By that point it was one of my least embarrassing episodes.

Two men in white lab coats were there. One was looking at my X-rays. The other one was speaking with Mom—he introduced himself to me as Larry Einhorn.

"So this is the musician I've heard so much about," he said. "I was telling your mother that Dr. Ranalli has done nothing but sing your praises."

"I could say the same to you," I said.

Dr. Einhorn was even shorter than me. Crooked wire spectacles were balanced on his nose. He was a non-creepy Woody Allen.

He looked nothing like I thought he would, but exactly like I thought he should—he just straight-up *looked* like a genius.

The other man was Dr. Redding—the surgeon. He was handsome, about my parents' age. He shook hands harder than I'd have liked.

Dr. Einhorn and Mom discussed the highs and lows

of my treatment. He brought up some late-onset issues I needed to stay cognizant of. I had a hard time focusing—a conversation that would have once horrified me now sounded like nothing but small talk.

But it wasn't long before he got to the surgery.

"As you know," Dr. Einhorn said, "due to the size and progressed state of the mass at the time of Robert's diagnosis, Dr. Ranalli and I felt that a combination of both chemotherapy and surgical procedure would yield the best results. I'm especially pleased with the way Robert has responded to the therapy—his cancer markers are continuously down, and the mass has shrunk significantly. I can thankfully say it seems we've made the right decisions."

The room nodded in agreement.

"Dr. Redding and his team will be performing the operation. He is our top man here at IU, and has done similar procedures before."

Dr. Redding stepped forward.

"The mass seems to be isolated in the front of the chest cavity, directly in front of the right lung," he said. "As Larry just mentioned, the mass has shrunk significantly since the original diagnosis. I will do a frontal incision, so I can make sure the remaining mass is not wrapped around the tissue of the lung—if it is, there's a chance we may have to remove a small section of the lung, or perhaps an entire lobe. All that is unlikely. Less than a five percent chance, but there is only so much we can tell from the X-rays. I can't be positive until I get in there."

*   *   *

We drove back the same day and didn't make it home until one in the morning. I'd taken a double dose of promethazine—one of my nausea pills—to help me sleep. I got out of the car groggy and exhausted.

I walked up to the house. I wanted to take another pill, get in my bed, and sleep for a million hours.

I wasn't in bed for more than ten minutes before Nat woke me up.

He switched on my desk lamp. I moaned.

"*Shut up, dude.* I'm trying not to wake up Mom. She thinks I'm already asleep."

"So did I," I said, annoyed.

Nat sat on the side of my bed.

"Nah, fuck that. I was waiting till you got home. What did the doc say?"

"They said it's all good and they penciled my surgery in, for a couple days before you leave, actually."

"Damn. Weird."

"Fuck it. I'm glad. The sooner the better. I'm ready to get done with this bullshit."

"Me too, man," he said.

I reached for my glasses.

"Okay, motherfucker, let's see this tattoo."

"Well, be *quiet*. I'm trying to put off Mom's shit-fit as long as I can."

Nat held out his right arm. The entire thing was Saran-Wrapped. He slowly peeled it away as bright puddles of blood and ink pooled on the plastic.

He held the arm toward me.

A single tattoo covered nearly his entire arm, wrapping around above the elbow, all the way down to his hand.

The front of his arm was the midnight sky, the same one above the mountains surrounding us, and the sky was full of dark clouds and lightning. Near his elbow was a single star—it was bright red, like the ones on the map in the basement.

I took hold of his wrist and twisted his arm to see the inside.

The dark clouds broke open. Thick rays of yellow-orange light blazed through. A white-winged bird flew free above the storm. Around it were the words *Brothers Forever*.

The tattoo was huge, impossible to miss. The statement was simple and permanent. There, through the light and through the darkness, was a promise rendered fucking unbreakable.

SEVENTEEN

Skeleton Crew

1

The days came faster and faster. It was life on autopilot, a blank cycle of summer days and nights—every hour seemed to rush toward something more important than the present moment.

The band doubled up on rehearsals. From eleven until six, they played their setlist over and over. They played it backward. They played it in the dark. Nat obsessed over that nine-song, thirty-minute set.

His huge tattoo gave him some new punk rock authority over Brody and Doyle, who now looked less like equals and more like a half-assed entourage. They would practice for as long as Nat wanted. They would dress however he asked. Whatever it was, they would concede.

And dumb as it sounds, the tattoo on his arm gave me a sense of security. When he strummed his guitar and the ink hit the strings, I felt like I was still part of the music, still present.

Of course, my mom flipped out when she saw it. She was convinced he'd finally thrown his life away, and took it as some sort of personal insult, like Nat got tattooed just to spite her. All of a sudden, Mom got on his case about *everything.*

But Nat said it had nothing to do with the tattoo. He thought Mom was mad because he would be on tour while I had my surgery in Indianapolis.

But if she *was* upset about it, she never let it show around me.

I didn't see what the big deal was. Why did Mom care if Nat was in Indy? Did she expect him to rush into the operating room and help with the surgery? I mean, we all knew how fucked up everything was—one more person in a waiting room wasn't going to help anything.

But I had no idea what Nat thought of our situation. We never talked about it anymore. Not the surgery. Not the cancer. Not even the tour.

Now we only talked about the future. Our summer was nothing but a means to an end. All that mattered to us was the after.

2

Fourth of July was the last day that we were all together.

We went downtown to watch the fireworks. Just Nat, Paul, Ali, and me.

It felt like years since I'd gone down for the show. I remembered skateboarding down Fifth Avenue, weaving through honking cars and crowds of patriotic hillbillies and miners.

But this year, we walked.

Ali wore faded jean shorts and a Springsteen T-shirt.

A couple of drunks chanted "Born, in the U-S-Ayeeee" as we passed by. Small, shifting groups of people inched slowly down the sidewalks. Crew-cut families in cutoff shorts bought snow cones and piss beer from vendors. We were all headed down to the river.

The streets smelled like gunpowder. Streamers hung off lampposts in blue, white, and red. Fat children ran shirtless, holding burnt-out sparklers and cheap little American flags.

Most of the crowd was already gathered on the muddy banks of the river. A few climbed on top of the flood wall—a chick tossed a bottle to the train tracks below. The crowd stretched for blocks. Families hollered impatiently, ready to see fireworks.

They were all idiots.

The best place to watch was the bridge.

The Robert C. Byrd Bridge stretched right over the river—from downtown Huntington into Ironton, Ohio—any folks with half a brain walked onto the bridge to watch.

The four of us scored a place right against the dirty railing. I looked down at the water below.

It was almost dusk. The sun reflected off the catfish water in a way that made me feel homesick, although I didn't quite understand why. A barge loaded to blow was anchored in the middle of the river.

The first firework came without warning.

There was a sudden, high, whistling sound, and then . . . *BANG!*

Each explosion was louder than the one before it. The smoke and sulfur were heavy in the air. We yelled and clapped, first jokingly, then not. We howled over the bridge like animals, trying to outdo the cannon fire.

Everything was beautiful.

Even Huntington looked beautiful, frozen there in the glow of that fire. Everyone was smiling. Engines hummed free on the bridge behind us. The river curled in brightly colored waves as the sky exploded both above and below us. I was somewhere in the middle of it all, the whole world on fire and me untouched.

It was a summer night in Shitsville, and everything was fine. I knew it then, as sure as I knew anything—it was almost over. I was going to be just fine.

EIGHTEEN

This Nightmare Place

1

Two days before I left for Indianapolis, three days before Nat left for tour, the front-page headline of our local paper read APPLEBEE'S COMES TO DOWNTOWN HUNTINGTON!

Getting a chain restaurant in our town was huge. There were fucking billboards and everything. So before we started our journey west, we stopped there for lunch on the way out of town. Nat drove to the restaurant separately, since he was staying behind.

He and I sat together on one side of a booth, and our parents sat on the other. None of us spoke. We chewed the microwaved food in silence, each of us lost in our own thoughts.

I was thinking of Ali.

She'd stopped at the house to say goodbye. She brought me her rosary, with a crucifix and beads of hand-carved wood. I put it in my backpack with the rest of my good-luck charms—my hospital cross, my picture Bible, Ali's Catholic shit, a Defiance of Authority button and a copy of our demo, a few paperbacks, and the first Pennywise cassette I ever bought.

I packed my toiletries, chemical mouth rinse, and two sets of clothes. I wrote *FUCK CANCER* on the tips of my Converse with a Sharpie before I put them in the backpack. The rest of the bag was filled with childproof prescription bottles.

Now the backpack leaned against my leg, as I sat in the restaurant waiting for someone to speak. No one did. The waitress cleared our plates. She brought the check.

It was time to go.

The four of us stood in the parking lot. The sky was overcast. Nat wore his sunglasses anyway.

Dad gave him a one-armed hug and a stiff pat. He took some twenties out of his pocket and handed them to Nat.

"For gas," he said.

Mom hugged Nat *hard*. Her shoulder blades moved quickly with her breath. She held on to him for a long time and she whispered something that I couldn't make out, kissed him on the cheek, and surrendered him.

He wiped her lipstick from his face. Mom and Dad walked to the car, leaving Nat and me standing alone.

We must have looked strange to the cars pulling in—a tattooed, black-clad rocker in Wayfarers and this pale, odd-looking bald boy beside him.

"Well," I mumbled, "I guess just let me know how the shows go."

He nodded. "Let me know how it goes in Indy."

I nodded.

We stared at the ground. We didn't cry. We didn't hug.

We didn't even shake hands. We just stood there, surrounded by cars. No goodbye seemed to fit.

Dad honked the horn.

"Well, I guess see ya."

Nat smiled sadly. "Later, bro. Later."

2

Dad booked two rooms at the Doubletree near University Avenue. It was the nearest hotel to the hospital. We needed to be close as I was due at 7 a.m. for "pre-op."

I was in Room 646. Mom and Dad were 648. They dropped off their bags and went for a drink at the bar. Mom told me I could get room service.

I'd never had my own hotel room before. The bed could have fit all three of us. The pillows were expensive foam. The window took up the whole wall.

I called the front desk. I ordered a cheeseburger and two sides of fries. When she said that they only served *unsweet* tea, I really felt far from home.

I picked at my food. I wasn't hungry. I had the TV on—some western on AMC—I wasn't paying attention. I kept it on for the noise. For the company.

How many people had watched this TV, slept in this bed, pissed in this toilet—hundreds, thousands? All these people passed through the same place, and there wasn't even a trace of them left.

Businessmen. Whores. Actors. Cops. Housewives. Children. Mothers. Different people leading different lives. Each just *gone* with no sign that they'd ever even been here at all. . . .

I looked out the window. I leaned my head against the glass. I wanted the smudge to stay there forever. I didn't want to be tidied up.

I thought about calling Nat but didn't. I wondered if he was ready to go. I wondered how much film Paul packed for his camera. I hoped Doyle remembered to bring enough drumsticks.

There was a knock at the door.

It was Dad. He grabbed a handful of fries from my tray and shoved them in his mouth.

"You better eat this stuff," he said. "The doc said no food or drink after ten tonight."

"I'm good."

He shrugged.

"Is Mom still at the bar?" I asked.

"Nah, we weren't down there ten minutes before she went back to the room. She wanted to double-check your prescription lists again before tomorrow and make sure the docs here know everything you're on. She brought all her notes and shit—you know how your mom is."

"I definitely do."

"Don't let her freak you out, it's going to go fine. You're a lot tougher than you give yourself credit for."

"I don't know about that," I said, embarrassed. No one had ever called me tough before.

He hugged me and his arms felt massive around my shoulders. Or maybe I just felt small.

* * *

The alarm clock startled me awake—five thirty.

I showered. I dressed. I wondered how I was supposed to take my medication if I couldn't drink anything.

I put on my *FUCK CANCER* Chucks. I said a half-assed prayer to Ali's rosary and then threw it in the bag with the rest of my shit.

I sat on the bed in the empty half dark. I turned on the TV. I turned it off. I stared out the window. I stared at my feet.

My parents knocked. They stood in the hall with their bags. They didn't look like they'd slept.

"Let's get this done with," Mom said.

I took one last look at the dark room. I sighed and followed them down the hall.

* * *

After I checked in and put on my gown, the nurse led me to my hospital bed. The sheets were freezing. She began my IV. The nurse injected two syringes into the tube, some heavy-duty shit that she promised would help me relax. I wished she had given some to my parents too.

The nurse left us. I started to feel the injections kick in. *Relaxed* isn't the right word for how I felt—*detached*, maybe. I felt like I was nervous somewhere inside, but the medications had mercifully muted that part of my brain.

Dr. Redding came down the hall to greet us.

He looked rested and confident. He rehashed the procedure briefly and then left to go prepare. My parents said he was a nice man.

A nurse came with paperwork. They wouldn't let Mom sign anymore, since I was eighteen. I tried to read it. The words blurred together, but I signed the papers anyway.

Twenty minutes later, they came for me.

Dad and Mom leaned over the bed and hugged me. They both said they loved me. I took off my glasses and handed them to Mom. She bent down again and kissed my bald head.

"Call Nat and tell him how it goes," I told her.

She nodded. She didn't say anything more.

Strangers in white wheeled me away.

* * *

The operating room was as huge and bright as a movie set. I counted ten people inside, all sheathed in full-body suits made of blue paper. A giant light hung on a movable arm above the center of the room. There was another bed beneath it. The operating table, I guessed.

The orderlies lifted me from my bed and put me on the table. It was cold. They wrapped an extra blanket around my legs. Then they had me lean up so they could undo my gown and lower it down to my chest.

It wasn't until that moment that I actually considered the fact that there was a tangible thing inside of me. The drugs and the side effects were one thing—but this wasn't as simple as an illness. All of a sudden, I understood that

I was about to have something hard and real and living carved from the middle of my chest.

My heart rate increased. Someone gave me another injection.

Dr. Redding asked me how I was feeling. Fine, I said. I couldn't read his expression through the face mask. Another blue-paper person fitted an oxygen tube into my nostrils and a clear plastic mask over my mouth.

"Okay, Robert, just count backward from ten in your head."

I nodded—*okay*. I started counting.

Ten, nine, eight . . .

(Soon I would be able to breathe again . . .)

. . . seven, six, five, four . . .

(Soon this horrible thing inside me would be . . .)

. . . *three, two* . . .

(Gone.)

3

I scream when I wake, but there is no sound.

The scream is inside my head, a high-pitched panic like twisting metal. There is a pressure in my throat—*somethingsomeone is choking me!*—I bite down and realize something has been shoved into my throat. I shake my head madly, gagging on the object.

Panic envelops me.

I try to cough it up but only swallow the object deeper. I claw at my mouth—there is a wide, ridged tube stuck down my throat.

I pull at the tube wildly, gripping and thrashing like I'm

trying to strangle it. Pain fills my body as the tube *rips* up from deep in my guts, through and out my throat. I pull it from my mouth. Bloodspit flecks spill onto my chest.

I gag. Everything is white and out of focus.

Alarms and buzzers sound. My eyes roll around in my head. I can't see or understand what is happening. I sense others near me, but they are blurred ghosts.

Just as I sit up, I feel two pairs of hands behind me, pushing me back on the bed. My arms are pinned back. I look down.

For the first time I see myself—this time when I scream, I can hear it perfectly.

Panic.

Now I am choking for real, inhaling empty, useless breaths of air. People move all around me.

"Can't you do something? *Can't you do something?*" someone shrieks. I know it is my mother, though I don't recognize the voice.

She leans over me, clutching my bedrail. Her eyes are bloodshot red and blue. She grabs my hand. Her nails *dig* into my skin.

Someone injects me with something. I try to breathe, but I can't.

The tension in my body grows weak. My hand goes limp inside my mother's hand.

She fucking *howls.*

"*They took your lung!*" she yells, unable to control herself. "*Ohgodjesuschrist oh nonono! They took it they took your heart they took your lungs oh no ohgodgod!*"

"Shut the fuck up!" I hear my father scream. She is pulled away from me with such force that the bed moves with her.

My consciousness begins fading from the room.

Mom is just confused. She didn't mean me.

Shadows of people move all around me. I can see sunlight, glowing somewhere through a window behind them.

Then nothing.

4

I am scared and lost. I hurt in a hurt that I never knew was possible.

I wake in short, distorted pockets. The first thing that registers, every single time, is the tube still jammed down my throat. I don't know what it does or why. I don't know where it goes.

Other tubes go under the blanket of my hospital bed. They must attach to me—my body can't feel enough for me to know.

Whenever I stir, they inject me. I don't ever wake for long.

Consciousness is a relative term in this nightmare place. I feel like I'm not even truly here. I am cut up. Ripped up. I don't understand what happened to me, or this constant pain—only that drugs keep it farther away.

So they keep me doped up. Thank God I am doped up. I know there are others like me in rooms like mine. I heard screaming earlier, though it may have been inside of a dream.

No part of me cares that I am still alive.

*   *   *

It is daytime when they remove the tube from my throat. The tube was breathing for me, they say. Now I must breathe on my own.

Mom is here. She is silent now. She sits in the corner near the window. Dad stands straight, his hands braced on the back of a chair.

A doctor pulls the tube through my insides and out of my throat. The pain crashes in my chest like lightning over the morphine cloud.

I *gasp* for air. It feels thin and useless.

I try to speak, but the pain is too much. My throat is as dead and hot as a desert.

They take the tube away. I see blood. Someone places a straw in my mouth. My *gasps* pull water in—the thin stream trickling down my throat makes me wince.

* * *

A male nurse shakes me awake.

"I need to change your bandages," he says.

He looks at my parents. "You may want to leave the room."

They walk out into the hall.

The nurse has stripped me to my waist. There is a giant white gauze pad covering my chest. Below, there are two thick rubber tubes bandaged to my sides. I try to ask him what they are. My throat hurts too much for sound.

"They're drainage tubes," he says, as if reading my mind. "They remove the fluid after the surgery."

I feel him ease the tape around the gauze off my hairless pigskin chest. I feel a tug—*painful*. Finally, I look down at my chest again.

I instantly want to vomit.

A dark-red knife gash, a quarter inch thick, stretches all the way across the width of my chest. The cut curves up beneath my nipples, which flop dejectedly over it. The red skin is clamped together with twenty thick staples; each caked in the shit-brown crust of dried blood.

I begin to gag.

The nurse sighs sympathetically. Gently, he cleans the blood from the staples with a damp cloth. I can't watch.

If I don't see it I can't feel it if I can't feel it I won't see it.

I shut my eyes. Tears leak out through the cracks.

I open my eyes. He has changed the bandage. I see the blood-soaked gauze sitting idly on the edge of my bed.

Now he removes the gauze around the tube sticking out from my left rib. This tube isn't going out, it's going *in*—sewn to my skin with a thick black thread. I see my stomach muscles tense. The tube moves with them.

There is no blood around this wound, just a yellow-pink ring of pus. The nurse wipes it away. He applies a fresh dressing. Then he moves to the tube on the other side of my stomach.

I don't want to watch anymore.

*   *   *

This room is different than the rooms on the cancer ward. There are no children here. The nurses move unsympathetically in and out, in and out. In this place there is no sympathy. No kids, no gods, no illness. Here there is only this pain. And thin streams of air.

Every inch of me aches. I long for the cancer ward in Ohio. I pray to be sick and puking and miserable, anything but in this pain.

I know that I am somewhere in Indiana. I shut my eyes and try to imagine the country surrounding me. The cornfields, rippling like black waves in the night. The stars above them—*endless* stars, carelessly shining like sparklers on the Fourth of July. I bet they look pretty outside this room.

But it doesn't matter. Eventually, the pain covers all.

NINETEEN

The Summer That Was

1

They began weaning me off the morphine.

It was harder this time. My pain was all-consuming, even with the drugs. Now, it became more present every day. *I* was more present too.

Dr. Einhorn came to see me many times, but I was unaware of it. I do remember Dr. Redding. My first clear thoughts were of him explaining again what had happened during the surgery.

When they opened my chest up, they discovered that the cancer had progressed further than they'd expected. Although it had significantly shrunk, the tumorous mass in my chest was *gigantic*—heavier than both of my lungs, combined—and its black roots were wrapped around my other vital organs like tentacles.

Dr. Redding performed an unprecedented, six-hour surgery.

He worked around my other organs, removing as much of the tumor as he could. But the mass was so big, so *enveloped* over my organs that, in the end, he decided it would be riskier to leave the tainted sections inside me than to remove them completely.

So, after the surgeon removed the tumor, he went to work removing a large section of my inferior vena cava (the vein that carries blood to my heart). They removed half of my diaphragm. They removed my entire right lung.

They restructured my chest cavity into a jumbled series of pins, rods, and meshing. My heart was now in the center of my chest. My remaining lung now shifted in the empty space. Mesh walls were attached to replace my missing diaphragm and keep my intestines from floating up into my chest.

Then they stapled me back together.

The tube in my throat forced my new body to breathe. The tubes in my ribs sucked the fluid and poison from the now-barren parts of my insides.

I didn't know how to process the information.

I wanted more drugs *now*.

I had been so certain I'd be breathing normally again once the tumor was gone. Now, the chances of that were fucking ripped away. Dr. Redding said they'd begin daily pulmonary-function tests, to measure how well my new body was adapting. Right now, my breathing capacity was down to twenty-three percent.

He said that it would get better.

"Will . . . I be able to . . . play drums again?" I choked out, before Dr. Redding left the room.

He looked at me, pathetic in bed.

"You need to focus on getting your strength back. You haven't eaten anything in five days, Robert. Your body has been through a *lot*. It needs energy. When you're strong enough, we need to get you walking again. You won't leave the hospital until you can walk. So let's focus on getting you home, and then we can work our way up to drums."

I still didn't eat. Food was impossible. It hurt too bad to take my pills. And unless I was complaining, it hurt too bad to talk.

Talking also would mean I'd have to talk about what happened, which might cause me to let go of some of the rage I was feeling. And I wasn't ready to do that. Not yet. The rage was the only feeling I could understand. So I held it in, clinging to it like it was a life preserver or a friend.

*　　*　　*

A doctor came into my room the next day. I didn't recognize her. A nurse and two very large male orderlies followed. The doctor was cheery. She smiled broadly over the turtleneck rising from her lab coat.

"It's finally time to take out those drainage tubes," she said warmly.

My breath caught in my throat—I felt way too *here* for this.

"Don't I need to get put to sleep?" I was requesting, more than asking.

"No, no," she said, "nothing like that. This is simple. We can do it right here—it'll only take a moment."

"Can I at least have some numbing stuff, or pain medicine? They're sewn inside me, right?"

She took the chart from the end of my bed. She flipped through it. She shook her head.

"Normally *yes*, but not for you. Sorry. They're trying to get you off that bad ol' stuff."

"Is it going to hurt?" I asked softly.

She thought it over. She smiled again and then shrugged.

"I guess it depends—some patients don't think it hurts too bad. Then again, some patients say that it's the worst pain they've ever experienced. . . ."

Before I could respond, the two orderlies held my arms to the bed. The nurse removed my blanket and lowered my gown. The doctor took a pair of nine-inch metal shears from her coat pocket.

"Jesus! Fuck!" I yelled. I squirmed. My chest hurt. The shears glistened. . . .

"Hold the left one, please," the doctor said flatly.

The nurse pinched my skin, below the suture. The shears made a metal-on-metal sound as they opened. The doctor quickly snapped the skin that was sutured around the tube completely *off*.

She yanked the tube out—it was *loooong*—and I gasped as I felt it move inside my insides, through the muck of my organs and blood until it finally came out of the hole in my stomach in one unnatural slurp.

My mouth was frozen open in shock.

The doctor immediately sewed it shut. Then she cut the second tube. I felt it thrashing through my insides like a fishing lure.

It was the worst pain I ever experienced.

* * *

They brought me Jell-O. Maybe my throat hurt too bad to eat real food—but this wasn't real food. This was J-E-L-L-O.

It was green. Why the fuck would they bring me green? Nobody likes green.

"You *have* to eat it," Mom said.

She and Dad sat together, barely looking at each other. I stared at the Jell-O cup on the rolling tray before me.

"Fuck that," I grumbled. "Not. Hungry."

"Well, you want to get outta here, don't you?" Mom said. "I sure know I do. I know that your dad does too. They won't let you leave until you start eating."

I finally picked up the spoon.

Even that small movement made my chest hurt. I brought a spoonful of green to my mouth. I let it linger on my tongue before it slid down my ravaged throat.

I'd been afraid that they might have hooked my insides up wrong. I was afraid that if I ate, soon Jell-O would be floating around inside of me forever.

I braced myself. Nothing happened.

I picked the spoon back up. The Jell-O (even this bullshit green) tasted amazing. I finished the entire cup.

I asked Mom if she could find me some more—preferably red. Mom clapped and ran out into the hall.

Once she was gone, Dad sat his paperback down in his lap. He looked at me squarely.

"You know what Redding said, about you getting your breath back? About drumming?"

"Yeah."

"Well, the body has ways of making up for missing organs. People who lose kidneys, for instance—that other kidney picks up the slack. Your lung will be no different. It might take a while, but I'm sure your breathing will get back to normal."

"Seriously?" I asked.

"I don't see why not. Shit, there was a guy who used to pitch for the Reds—can't remember his name—but *he* only had one lung, and he ran those bases faster than any guy on the field. If he can play sports, you've got to figure that you can play drums."

"Are you making that up? That sounds—"

"*Listen*—do you want to be able to play drums again?"

I nodded.

"Okay, good—then you will. Case closed. You will."

*　　*　　*

They sent the same male nurse to get me—it was time for me to walk.

But first, I had to stand up. It took both him and my parents to steady me as my feet dangled over the floor. I eased one foot down slowly. They held on to my upper arms and helped me forward.

Soon, I had both feet on the cold floor. I took a shallow breath and eased all my weight down. My chest and back hurt, but not much worse than when I was in bed. The nurse hooked my catheter bag to the bottom of my IV stand.

"Your first challenge is walking to the bathroom," he said. "If you can make it there, I *might* be able to talk 'em into taking out that cath."

Fuck you, a voice inside hissed. *Fucking shithead fucking nurse prick I don't have to do it I don't have to listen to you fuck this fuck this place. . . .*

"Let's do it," I said.

I took ten pathetically small, incredibly slow steps forward—I was already out of breath. My gasps were shallow and scared. He told me to take my time, to relax, to *breathe.*

But breathing felt so strange. The air flowed into my mouth the same, but then it seemed to get lost somewhere inside me.

"You just gotta get used to it," the nurse said. "You gotta let your body get reacquainted with itself. You know?"

I nodded again. I took eight more baby steps forward.

Twenty-three minutes and forty-one steps later, I was inside the bathroom.

"Yeah," the nurse said. "Good job! Now catch your breath, and we'll try to make it back to the bed."

"Cool . . ." I panted, ". . . let's . . . do . . . it."

*　　*　　*

The next day, he had me walk to the hallway.

The catheter was gone. No breathing tube, no drainage tubes, no piss tube—I was losing tubes every day. I was once again more man than machine.

I gripped my IV stand and inched down the hall, stopping every few feet. The nurse narrated as we walked, telling me about the patients in each room we passed.

This guy—six gunshots. Six! Room four, right there—motorcycle accident. Keep walking. . . . You don't need to see that.

The walking was murder on my body. I was still in

numbingly constant pain. I labored to breathe air that felt as useless as quicksand in my throat. But the more I learned about my Intensive Care floor-mates, the harder it was to feel sorry for myself.

Room eight, right next door to ya—burn victim. Third degrees on eighty-five percent of his body. Can you believe that? You think you're in pain, but burn victims are the worst. Imagine every single nerve ending you have frying, twenty-four hours a day. Nothing can help that guy, except maybe a bullet to the head.

Trust me, you don't wanna see him. Keep walking.

I kept walking.

*   *   *

Every day got a little better. Lack of movement gave me bedsores, so I had to rotate from bed to chair, chair to bed, just like I did on the cancer ward. I progressed from eating Jell-O to soup, then up to a few bites of chopped salad.

One day, a psychiatrist showed up at the room. She was young, and pretty-ish. Instead of a lab coat, she wore a tight blazer and tight pants. My parents left us alone in the room. She sat down casually across from my bed.

"So how are you feeling?"

"Fine, I guess," I said, "considering."

She nodded sympathetically. "You've been through quite a lot."

"Yeah."

"That's why I came to speak with you today, Robert. Many times when someone loses, say, an *arm*, they go through a transitional period of grief, not unlike when one loses a loved one. Do you understand?"

"Okay."

"Now, I know you didn't lose an arm, but those feelings of grief and depression are still very common in these cases."

I didn't say anything.

"May I ask—have you been feeling depressed"—*yes*—"or hopeless?" *Yes.*

"Not really."

"No?" she asked.

"Nope."

"Okay. What about feelings of anger"—*definitely*—"or anxiety"—*of course*—"since you've been here?"

"No more than what would be normal," I said, "*considering.*"

"That is interesting. Your caregivers have been concerned—that's why I came to visit today. Do you think you might be willing to try an antidepressant while you adjust?"

Yes, I thought.

"No," I said.

She smiled. She wished me luck.

*   *   *

Two days later, a nurse told me that I'd be discharged soon. I was surprised—I still felt nowhere *near* recovered. My walks were progressing, but slowly. My pulmonary numbers had barely improved.

"Honestly," the nurse said, "we need the space in the

ICU for other trauma patients. Compared to others on this floor, you are making *great* progress."

"Makes sense," Dad said.

"You'll be moved out of ICU and into a more comfortable room for a few days. After that, it shouldn't be long until your discharge goes through."

"All right," I said. Though I definitely wasn't feeling too excited about it.

The nurse smiled a sad smile. She looked out the window, into the sun. She put her hands on her hips and shook her head.

"My, my, my," she said, "have you guys had a hard one. Your family sure has a story, though—people won't know what to think when you tell them about the summer that was . . ."

She paused, searching for a word to finish her thought. She never found it.

2

They moved me into the nicest hospital room I'd ever seen. It was three times the size of a normal room. The floor was carpet, not cold tile. There was a large TV with cable, a couch, and a window. The bed was actually comfortable.

At first, I didn't notice that they'd gotten me a room in the hospice. Later, they would say that it was the only free bed in the building.

This wasn't like the hospice I'd imagined in the children's hospital. This wasn't so bad at all. If some old fuck was forced to die in a hospital, there were worse rooms than this to do it in. The change in scenery lifted my spirits a little. The move put me that much closer to home.

A few times a day, a nurse made me do a breathing test using an incentive spirometer—an empty plastic measuring container with a tube on the end. You blow in the tube. When you exhale, the force of your breath moves a measurement dial.

I hated doing it.

Not because it was hard, but because the nurse pushed me, and *pushed* me—I'd move the dial halfway up, and she would tell me to do better. I'd exhale again—halfway up. She'd again say, "Do better."

"Jesus, lady," I finally said. "I just . . . got my lung . . . removed, I . . . think I'm doing pretty . . . good. . . ."

She nodded. "Oh, you are! Now do *better*."

*   *   *

It was alone in the hospice that I finally decided to call Nat. We hadn't talked at all. My parents hadn't mentioned him.

I tried his cell—he answered.

"Yo!" he said, excited. "How are you feeling, man?"

"Eh," I mumbled, not sure how to answer. "Not as bad as I was. How is tour going?"

"*Amazing!* I wish you were here, bro."

"Me too. You get to meet any other bands yet?"

"I met Tim Armstrong from Rancid yesterday— *backstage*," he said proudly.

"*Whoa*. What did he say?"

"Not a lot, really. He was walking backstage, and I bumped into him when I was carrying my amp to the van. He told me to get the fuck out of his way."

"Damn!" I said. "That's so rad."

"Yeah, it was pretty badass. So how is your breathi—"

"Where are you guys at tonight?" I asked quickly. I didn't want to talk about my breathing.

"A Super 8, outside of Philly. We had the day off, decided to stop here tonight."

"Is Philadelphia cool?"

"We went downtown an hour ago and got cheesesteaks," he said. "They put fucking *Cheez Whiz* on them, dude."

"Fuck. Gross."

"Kinda, but the city seems okay. Day after tomorrow is Cleveland—it's the last show of the tour." He sighed. "I never imagined I'd be beating you home."

"No shit," I said. "I wish I was gonna be in Philly, or even Cleveland. And you know I hate Ohio."

"Me too," he said. "Me too. . . ."

Someone called for him in the background. He hissed at them to *hold on.*

"You got a window in that hospital room?" he asked.

"Yeah, they moved me to a new room. It's legit."

"Did you see the moon? It's fucking huge tonight."

I eased over to the window. I covered the receiver as I struggled for breath. The moon *was* huge—it was an orangish-copper color, a moldy tangerine in the sky.

"I see it."

"Good," he said, "me too. If you can see it, and I can see it, maybe we really aren't that far away."

"Yeah. Maybe not."

It was in that way we said good night.

I called Ali next.

I was so thankful she wasn't there to see me laid up. The call was dramatic enough.

To keep it light I asked her what she'd been up to since I'd been gone. I should have just told her about the surgery instead.

"I don't know. Just *stuff*. Whatever," she mumbled.

"Uh, all right," I said. "You okay, babe?"

"I'm fine."

Girls are so fucking weird.

"You don't sound fine," I said.

She sighed. "It can wait until later."

"What can?"

"Nothing."

"Ali—you're a horrible liar, and you know it. Just tell me what's going on."

"I—[*sniffle*]—told myself I wasn't gonna tell you until after."

"Tell me *what*?"

"Well, it wasn't my fault," she said. "Let me just say that first."

"Okay," I said. My body tensed.

"I went to a party last weekend, with Mandy. At Adam's place."

"Okay."

"Well, so everyone was there and there was tons of booze and I've been so stressed out lately—with your surgery, and money, and school starting again soon—so I got like, pretty wasted."

"Okay."

"Well, like I got *blackout* kinda wasted. And you know Teddy, my boyfriend before the boyfriend before the guy I was dating right before you?"

"Yes."

"Well, he showed up. *He* was blackout drunk too, and he started like, grabbing all over me, right in front of everyone."

". . ."

"Nothing really happened. I don't think. I was *so* fucking drunk, Rob. But I am, like, pretty positive nothing happened. Okay? I just wanted to tell you before someone else started gossiping about it, or something."

The world turned *red*.

I had to get off the phone—*now*.

"I have to go," I snapped. "Sorrytalktoyoulaterbye."

I slammed down the receiver. It didn't help.

I threw the phone at the wall. My wound *throbbed*.

A nurse rushed in.

"What happened?" she asked.

"I need medicine. I am in serious pain."

3

When I woke, the sun was in my eyes, reflecting off the blank TV screen. I got up slowly. I walked shakily into the bathroom. Balancing against the wall, I grabbed the geriatric rails around the toilet.

Godfuckingdamn, I hurt.

I pushed myself off the toilet. I eased to the sink. I

glanced up at the mirror and looked at my bandaged chest. Half the dressing had come off as I slept. I could see the corner of the wound. It looked as raw as uncooked hamburger. I cringed. My gut tightened.

But that's when I saw it—*hair!*

Not a lot—shit, barely enough to count, just a shadow of hair. Little buds of stubble popped up around my ears and the top of my head.

I ran my hand over it—I *felt* it! The skin was rough, like used sandpaper. I brushed my hand over my head—*over my hair*—again, laughing like an idiot at my own reflection.

* * *

I could walk down the entire hallway now. It still took forever, and I still had to stop a lot—it was walk, break, breathing test, walk, break, breathing test—but I now had the confidence to keep going. I wanted to do better.

And I was.

Mom told me that they were going to let me leave in the next day or two. I still didn't feel ready to be discharged—I could barely breathe, and I was still in pain. I wanted to go home, but I also knew what home *meant*—that the rest of my recovery was up to me.

I called Nat again that night, on the new phone the orderly brought. He told me the show in Jersey ruled; that it was the biggest crowd he'd ever played to. He said he couldn't wait for *us* to go back and play there again.

He asked me if I'd talked to Ali yet. I told him about the party. About Teddy. I couldn't help it. He listened to the story in complete silence.

"When did this happen?" he finally said.

"Last weekend, I think."

"Do you know Teddy's number?"

"Nah." Then, embarrassed, I added, "But I bet Ali still does."

He sighed. "Jesus. Okay, thanks. See you at home."

The line died.

* * *

Two days later, the word came down—I was finally going home.

The nurse said I could take a shower, but that also meant cleaning my own wounds. She brought me a towel, along with packages of gauze, medical tape, and huge white bandages.

I was afraid to let the water touch my incisions. I stood under the showerhead with my back toward it and my chin bent down. I covered my chest and let the warm water wash over the tops of my shoulders. I ran my hand over my head, savoring the roughness of it.

Mom helped me dress my wounds. Our nurse gave me a bottle of painkillers and more bandages. My chest was too sore for me to put on a T-shirt, so I had to borrow one of Dad's button-ups. It was loose on my body and barely touched my skin.

No doctors came to see me off. No nurses came to tell us goodbye. An orderly showed up outside my door with one of those beautiful wicker wheelchairs.

I sat down in it. The orderly let Dad roll me to the car. I made it out of the hospice, alive.

*   *   *

I took two painkillers before we even got to the car. Mom opened the door for me, and I lay slowly in the backseat, using my backpack for a pillow. I asked Dad to ride easy.

It was late afternoon when we pulled out of the hospital parking lot. It was already August. The summer was already done.

Dad's yelling woke me up. I rubbed my eyes and looked toward the front seat. He was on his cell phone. When he hung up, I asked what was wrong.

"Oh, I don't know," he said sharply. "Maybe your goddamn knucklehead of a brother, or your idiot buddy Paul can tell you."

"Nat?" Mom said. "What about him?"

"Well, that was my buddy from the police station. He called to let me know that someone in *our* neighborhood just called the cops on *your* son."

"What?" we both said.

"Apparently he and Paul assaulted someone, a few blocks from the house."

Mom put her face in her hands.

"There's no way," I said from the backseat. "Who called the cops?"

"Reed, something."

Shit.

"Teddy Reed?"

"Do you know him?" Dad said. He looked back at me.

"Kind of."

At that exact moment, the strangest thing happened.

A family of deer stood on the empty highway ahead of us—six of them, unmoving, in between the rows of corn. Dad wasn't paying attention and he didn't have time to brake.

We plowed right fucking into them.

Mom screamed. I flew forward, hitting my chest hard against the back of the seats. I lay on the floor moaning, straining to get up.

Dad didn't even slow down.

"Fuck it," he said. "This car's a piece of junk, anyway."

I crawled back onto the seat and looked out the rear windshield—a deer lay dying, twitching on the cement. The other deer still stood there, gathered around the injured one. They didn't move. They watched over him hopelessly, there on the empty road.

TWENTY

Prodigal Son/Weeping Saint

1

The tour van was parked in front of the house when we arrived. It was just sitting there, like it had never left. Déjà vu again and again. Everything changes but remains the same.

I stared at the concrete steps leading to our yard. I hadn't progressed to stairs, yet here were eight of them, hard and chipped, and waiting for me.

I inched across the sidewalk toward them. I leaned on the railing to catch my breath.

"Shit . . ." I panted. "How . . . am I . . . supposed to do this?"

"One step at a time," Mom said from behind me. "The only way you can."

By the time I made it up the stairs I was exhausted. But *I made it up!*

I kept moving through the yard, afraid to lose momentum. I climbed the front porch . . . my chest heaved . . . I leaned onto the porch rail . . . Dad unlocked the door. . . .
Inside.

It was dark, and mercifully cold. I sat down on the couch, still trying to catch my breath. The lights were off. Nat must have been asleep.

The place smelled the same. I huffed the fumes of home. I didn't want to move.

I decided just to sleep there, on the couch. I didn't have the energy to walk upstairs to my bedroom.

Mom brought me blankets and a pillow. What I needed (*wanted*) was painkillers. She gave me the bottle. I took one, and then lay on the matted couch.

After I was settled, my parents marched to the basement door. They threw it open, flipped on the light, and stormed down. I heard Nat wake up. I heard them all start yelling. Welcome fucking home.

Through snippets of their argument, I pieced together the events of the night.

Nat and Paul decided to confront Teddy almost as soon as they got back into town. Nat tried calling his house first. He called again. And again. He left ten messages. Teddy never called back.

He called again—the phone was off the hook. So, the two of them decided to stop by his place. . . .

The Reed family lived in a big house, near the park. They had a gigantic yard that Teddy had turned into a makeshift soccer field. All Nat planned to do was tell him off, call him out. He knew that Teddy was at home—his car was parked right out front. But no one answered the door.

So they waited. They paced the porch. They got angry.

Nat *told* my parents the reason he went over there.

I could hear his voice from the basement, trying to explain. . . .

. . . This guy is man enough to try and screw my brother's girlfriend while he's in the hospital, but not man enough to answer the door?! So I started thinking, Screw THAT! And I just . . .

Nat said that they waited for a half hour, until his cell *finally* rang—it was Teddy's mom. She demanded Nat leave them alone.

Paul *pounded* on their door now, angrier than ever. No one would answer. Eventually, they decided to try another tactic.

A large bag of soccer balls was tied to the goalpost in the yard.

They started kicking soccer balls at the front door of the house.

They *aimed* for the front door, at least—but it wasn't like they had their own practice field at home.

Balls smashed potted plants. Balls chipped siding. Balls dented the gutter. A ball murdered a lawn gnome. Nat scored a *GOOOOAL*—straight through the fucking living room window.

That's when they saw police lights moving down the street.

They left the soccer balls and took off running. Nat cut through the alley, Paul ran toward the park. When they met at my house, two hours later, there were no police waiting to arrest them, no phone messages, no nothing. Nat had figured they'd gotten away with it.

Dad called him a fucking idiot.

He said he was lucky he wasn't arrested. He bitched

my brother out accordingly, but his tone wasn't harsh anymore. Mom's voice was too muffled to make out.

Their footfalls moved up the basement steps. They didn't tell him good night.

I felt responsible for all of it. When I told Nat about Teddy and Ali, I must have known he'd do something like that—I must have *wanted* him to do something like that, right? I probably hoped for something worse.

But I hadn't meant to cause more friction in my own family. Shit, my issues left my parents mentally and emotionally spent—and Nat had missed *so* much while he was on tour.

Now things were even worse.

My parents had this new, crippled version of their son. I took up even more room, caused even more stress, and stole even more time, *Jesus Christ*. They weren't equipped to take on the problems of *two* kids, not anymore. So, without even knowing it, Nat was on his own. He was now an adult, while I was once again a child.

I hurt too bad to think about that shit anymore. I leaned onto the coffee table and popped another painkiller. I let it dissolve a little under my tongue. Then I swallowed, and hoped to pass out quick.

2

I heard Nat in the kitchen when I woke. I groaned and sat up on the couch. My wounds felt sticky against the gauze. I must have sweated through the night.

I dragged myself into the kitchen.

Nat was at the table, drinking coffee with Mom. The scene was unexpected—I'd never seen him drink coffee, and the sight further confirmed his new aura of grown-upness. When he saw me he smiled.

"Yo man," he said, not getting up.

"Hey."

I winced when I sat down at the table. Mom brought me my morning meds and a glass of water. She sat the pills in front of me and then left the two of us alone.

Nat got up. He'd lost weight—he was almost as skinny as me. His hair was bigger. He wore ripped black shoes and jeans, and a sleeveless T-shirt. On his left shoulder was a new tattoo, a black-and-white vintage microphone. He looked like he didn't give a damn about *anything*. I wanted to look like that one day.

"Are you allowed to walk up and down stairs?" he asked.

"Yes, smart-ass."

"Then let's go down to the basement. I wanna show you what I brought you from the road."

"I'll meet ya down there," I told him. I didn't want him to see the way that I struggled.

When I finally got to the basement, my chest was throbbing in pain. I sat on the bottom step. Nat's suitcase was in the corner. It was still packed, like he was only visiting.

A Warped Tour backstage pass was sitting on the shelf beside his SIBLING ID card from Children's Hospital. I reached for the pass—it was just a piece of laminated plastic, faded a little around the sides. I had never played a show with backstage passes before—I'd never played anywhere with a *backstage* before! That dirty piece of plastic was eternally cool.

I put it back.

Nat leaned over his suitcase and started pulling stuff out. He laid the highlights of his adventures on me—seeing Jimmy Eat World in Asbury Park, right beside the ocean—when the singer of 7 Seconds watched their set from side stage—seeing AFI play different songs every day. He spoke of driving the Jersey Turnpike death-race, where the skyscraper horizon gleamed as sharp as switchblades. He described Pennsylvania forests, reaching higher and farther than ours ever could.

"And the girls. *Shit*, man. *The girls.*"

I laughed. "Whatever. Rock 'n' roll groupies died out with Def Leppard, bro."

"Dude, you have no idea. There were *so* many chicks at these shows! And, like, they'd come and talk to *us*! It was fucking insane. I met this one, in Louisville, who looked like Rachel Leigh Cook with a Mohawk."

"Have you talked to Ashley since you've been back?"

He looked annoyed. "Yeah. But she's been acting weird."

"Ashley always acts weird."

"Yeah, I know—but even her weirdness is getting weird. Whatever. Talking about that shit is a drag. Let me show you what I scored for you."

He brought tons of records and band shirts home for me, all autographed by the bands with phrases like *Stay up!* and *Get well soon, dude!* He brought me a Rancid beanie. AFI signed a drumstick for me. H2O gave me every piece of merch they had.

"I talked to the other bands about you a lot. By the time I left that tour, everyone knew your name, man."

"Trippy," I said self-consciously. I twirled the drumstick around in my hand—it had been months since I'd held one.

"I wish you could have been there," he said. "I wished it every fucking day."

"Forget it."

The room got quiet.

"So, how are you really feeling?" he asked.

"*Horrible.* I mean, I'm better than I was—but I'm in constant fucking pain, and getting so out of breath. That surgery, it messed me up bad, man."

Nat nodded. He asked to see my chest. I unbuttoned my shirt and labored at the soggy bandages. I clenched my jaw as I peeled them back.

"Shit," Nat said. "Brutal."

"You have no idea."

I tried to stick the bandages back on. Nat watched, unblinking.

"Thanks for going to Teddy's," I said, changing the subject.

Nat laughed. "Fuck that guy. Next time I see him, I'm gonna smash his face."

"Mom and Dad still pissed?"

"Nah, not really. You better call Paul, though—his mom lost her shit last night. The cops called their apartment, dude. She's threatening to send him to military school."

"You're kidding."

"Ah—don't worry about it. You know they don't have enough money to pay for some snooty-ass military academy."

"True," I said, "but still the whole thing is fucked."

"The whole *summer* was fucked, dude. We just gotta roll with it, same as we always do."

I nodded. I stood to go back up the stairs—and then, hopefully, up to my bedroom. I needed a shower. I needed to change my bandages.

I made it up three stairs, but then had to stop and catch my breath. My body just couldn't get used to working this way.

I leaned against the wall, panting.

"Whoa, whoa, shit, relax," Nat said. "Just chill a second, man. Don't rush it."

He leaned over and pressed play on the stereo. An old Rancid cassette was in the tape player. He cranked it up, shaking his head to the music.

"Man!" he yelled above the speakers. *"Do you remember how long ago we got this?"*

I remembered the exact moment—seeing the album cover, sitting on the rack of that faraway record store. Putting it on for the first time, back when we had no idea where it would take us . . .

. . . *He moved so slow, like a dying dream* . . .

* * *

I rested once more on the stairs, and then again at the kitchen sink. I was halfway to my room. I walked into our small foyer. I looked up at the stairs—twelve, steeper than the others. They might as well have been Mount Everest.

I sucked air and started climbing.

*   *   *

Dad showed up with an old TV from the pawnshop. He and Nat carried it up to my room. They hooked it up at the foot of my bed. I hoped that the mixture of pills and daytime TV could numb my brain enough for me to forget the pain—to forget about it all—if only for a little while.

I was watching a sitcom when Ali showed up.

I was lying there, on a stack of pillows. She stood at my door until I waved her inside. She moved toward me and held out her arms, but then paused. I told her it was fine, as long as she was gentle.

She gave me an awkward hug, kissed me on the cheek, and kneeled beside the bed. She smiled—the sad one—and rubbed her hand across my head.

"Holy shit, baby," she said, "your hair is growing back!"

"I know." I smiled. "I just hope it isn't curly."

"Can I see?"

"Sure," I said. I started to unbutton my shirt.

She gasped when she saw all the bandages. I asked her to help me unwrap the wounds. She peeled a bandage back. Her arm shook.

Even in the low light, the cuts looked vicious. The staples bit into the raw skin like razor fangs.

"Ohmygod," Ali mumbled.

She reached for the biggest cut but stopped. She closed her eyes, squeezing a few tears out, and took ahold of my hand. She lowered her head.

She just kneeled there silently, shaking her head with her eyes closed.

"Holy fucking shit," I said. "Seriously—you couldn't look more Catholic right now if you tried. Come on, Weeping Mary, get up. Get up, really, it's okay."

"Shut up, asshole." She laughed. She wiped her eyes.

She moved to the other side of the bed, and sat straight-backed beside me. We held hands and watched idiots laugh on TV.

Every few minutes, she asked me a question. Was I okay? When would I go back to Columbus? How was my breathing? Did I get to keep the lung? Was this almost *over*?

Vague answers were the best that I could do.

"Did you see Nat when you got here?" I asked her.

"No," she said quickly, her eyes fixed on the TV.

"Oh, well, he's down in the basement. You should have him tell you about—"

"About what? About Teddy? I already know *aaaaaallllllll* about it, Rob. Let's just *drop it*."

"What the hell is your problem?"

"After that shit your brother pulled the other night, *my* friends won't even *talk* to me! Everyone is pissed. And they're taking it out on me."

"So?" I said, after a moment. "So what if they don't talk to you? They suck. You *know* that they suck. Why would *you* want to talk to *them*? They shouldn't be mad at you, or my brother—or anyone but Teddy."

I couldn't believe I was hearing this shit. Her friends—all of whom *knew* I was in the hospital—weren't upset with Teddy. They were upset with me. They were upset that the events of their party didn't just fade away.

"But they're my friends, Rob," Ali said, softer now. "I mean, don't you get that? What do you want me to do? Hang out alone when you're gone? With only your brother, or Paul? I have to have friends. I *have* to have a life. *You know?* Don't look at me that way, Rob. Damn."

TWENTY-ONE

Skin-Deep

1

I *had* to get out of the fucking house.

For almost two weeks I stayed locked inside, barely moving, struggling and bitching to get from one room to another, but even I knew I needed to get out of bed. I needed to see if I could function in the outside world.

So Ali and I went to the movies. I took pain meds, and she offered to drive. She parked at the empty bank, a few blocks from the theater.

"Holy Christ," I said, as soon as I set foot on the blacktop.

"Yeah, it's been really hot this week. . . ."

Hot was an understatement. The dog-day weather turned our town into a fucking pressure cooker—the air was so thick I had trouble swallowing it. I labored through the parking lot, limping pathetically slow, posting on cars and brick walls for support.

"Should I take you home? This movie looks pretty stupid, anyway."

"I know it . . . does," I panted, "but we . . . are . . . fucking going . . . okay? Just . . . let me . . . catch my breath. . . ."

I strained to open the doors of the Keith-Albee The-ater. I felt a rush of calm as the cold air engulfed me. The lobby was empty, apart from the pimply kid at the box office. He said we were thirty-five minutes late for the movie.

"Give me . . . two tickets, anyway . . . man," I said. I handed him a twenty.

I bought popcorn for Ali and some Junior Mints for myself. With hope in my heart, I ordered a large Coke—if my hair was coming back, maybe my taste buds were too.

As I waited on my change, I heard someone say, *"Ali?"*

I turned toward the voice. There was a group of five frat guys at the ticket counter. One of them, the biggest, was waving.

She smiled and waved back. "Hey, James."

James walked over to her and gave her a hug. *James* wore a pastel-pink polo shirt and khaki shorts. *James* didn't ac-knowledge me, or even notice I was there. *James* made small talk, while Ali shuffled awkwardly.

Finally, his friends called for him. *James* walked the fuck away.

Ali helped me into the main theater.

"Who's James?" I whispered, as we walked past dark rows of seats.

"Just a guy I met at a party," she whispered back.

"I don't remember him from school. . . ."

"No, he's a junior at Marshall University."

"Awesome."

We sat in the front row.

I leaned back in my chair. I was still a little out of breath. I looked at the screen but couldn't pick up the story line. Dual thoughts raced down separate tracks in my mind—part of me kept saying, *Oh no, it took you half an hour to walk three blocks*—but the other part said, *Hell yes, you made it THREE BLOCKS!*

* * *

My wounds were looking better. They were turning lighter shades of red.

Our family doctor was back from his sabbatical and offered to remove the staples himself so that I wouldn't need to leave town. It didn't hurt as bad as I thought it would—he said it was because the nerves in my chest were probably all scrambled up.

But that wasn't important—the important thing was that the staples were out. The important thing was that slowly—*painfully* slowly—I was starting to work my way out of the trauma. The important thing was that, maybe, life could actually get back on track.

Nat was writing new songs. He'd written six brand-new ones while on the road, but he wouldn't let me hear them.

"Not yet," he kept saying. "Not until they are ready."

He wanted to have twelve new jams written and arranged by Christmas.

By Christmas, I'd be done with treatments, and my breathing would have hopefully improved enough for me to play drums again. By Christmas, everything would be cool. So we planned to arrange the new songs over winter break. By next spring, we would be ready to record a new demo, or maybe even a full-length.

"I'd really like to go ahead and do the band photo for the new press kit," I told him one day, "before I go in for those last chemo treatments. I don't really wanna be bald in the pictures."

Nat nodded. "I'll talk to Paul about taking some for us next week."

"Thanks. Hey, also, how long do you think I need to call in advance to make a tattoo appointment?"

"Shit, man, not long at all. You could probably call down there right now if you wanted. For you, the guys at the shop said anytime."

I called J-Sin's House of Ink later that afternoon. The counter girl put me on hold—when she came back, she told me that they were booked up for the entire month . . . but that Jason, the shop owner, would stay after they closed so he could squeeze me in.

"When?" I asked her.

"Tonight," she said. "Why dick around?"

Nat and I left the house around ten. We drove down darkened streets, toward the tattoo shop. It was the only place on the block with the lights still burning.

A hand-painted sign hung over the door—J-SIN'S HOUSE OF INK in melting black print. It swayed and creaked above me as I walked inside.

The door opened into a long hallway. The walls were painted with sugar skulls—a hundred black-and-white faces with folksy, thick-toothed grins. I followed the skulls down the hallway, past the waiting room, and into the first booth. Jason (J-Sin) sat on a rolling stool, waiting for me.

He was in a metal band that we played with sometimes.

He was about my height, but twice as wide. His cheeks were covered in surprisingly gray stubble. Faded tattoos curled around his arms and neck.

He told me to chill while he finished setting up.

He adjusted the gurney that spread across the length of the booth. He set an armrest to the left of it. He dropped colorful tears of ink into little plastic cups.

A stencil of Nat's tattoo sat on the counter beside him.

By the time he was ready, Paul, Ali, Doyle, Jamie, and Tyson were all there, showing support for my childhood dream of getting needles jammed into my skin. They cheered as I left the waiting room.

I lay on the gurney. Jason straightened my left arm onto the armrest. He shaved the arm with a safety razor. Not much hair had grown back yet, but he ran the blade down the skin just the same.

He called Nat back to the booth.

Jason took hold of Nat's right arm, straightening it beside mine. He pressed his stencil on my arm and evened it out with my brother's tattoo. He peeled off the paper, but the skeleton of the tattoo stayed.

With a red marker, Jason outlined the piece—the sky, the clouds, and the stars appeared in broad, sweeping lines. He repositioned my arm and then picked up his tattoo gun.

He tapped the pedal that controlled it—the gun went *bbbzzzzzzzz, bbz, bzz, bbzzzz bbbbbzzzzz*. It sounded like I was in a dentist's office, not a tattoo parlor. It sounded painful. . . .

"Ain't scared of needles, are you?"

I shook my head. "If I was, I'd know it by now."

He pressed his foot on the pedal, bringing the tattoo

gun back to life. Dozens of tiny needles moved on the tip of this torture device. He dipped the needles into the cup of black ink.

"Well, here we go," he said.

At first, there was only pressure—the sting of the needles was present, of course, but it wasn't like getting a shot, or a biopsy. These needles didn't puncture veins or bone. These needles went only skin-deep.

This is it? I wondered.

I relaxed as Jason drilled into my arm.

It wasn't it.

After three straight hours, I was in serious pain. The sting of the needles took on a raw quality as they treaded endlessly over old wounds. When Jason finally stopped for a smoke break, I was relieved.

He sprayed my arm with water, then dabbed off the extra ink and blood. He tossed the paper towel at the trash can but missed. Then he moved toward the front door, digging in his jeans for the smokes.

I dug around in my own jeans, searching for my pills. I placed a painkiller under my tongue and held it there. I walked to the bathroom, where I could stretch out my throbbing arm to get a real glimpse.

It looked *exactly* like Nat's tattoo. A matching red blood star shined farther near my elbow. I rotated my arm. I looked at it from all angles. The tattoo was almost finished. We were almost identical again.

I dipped my head beneath the bathroom faucet and swallowed the melting pill. Then I walked out to the waiting room to show everyone my progress.

"You should get tattooed while I recuperate," I said jokingly to Paul.

"Fuck it, I totally will."

Before I could reply, he was out the front door, standing on the stoop while Jason smoked his second smoke. I watched them talking through the window.

A few minutes later, Jason walked wordlessly past me. He went into the booth. Paul tore off his shirt and flung it at Ali.

"Hold my shirt, gorgeous," he said, and winked.

He followed Jason back.

It was like a fever spread through the House of Ink—in less than two hours, almost every one of us got tattoos. There was no forethought; Jason didn't even sketch them out anymore. He was working freehand, staying in the moment.

Paul got his back covered in red constellations. The stars grew darker as the blood pooled.

Tyson got a similar tattoo on his back, but without any thick outlines or shadow. It was like a watercolor—a painting of a giant storm cloud. Shots of lightning reached over the stars, curling like electric arms.

Doyle got the Black Flag logo tattooed onto his wrist.

"Me next," Nat said.

"Mom will kill you if you get another one."

"Eh, she won't notice," he said. "She doesn't even look at me, bro."

Jason yelled out from the booth: "Anyone else want a banger before I finish up Rob's sleeve?"

Nat walked past me, down the hall.

"Just a small one," I heard him say.

A few minutes later, the tattoo gun was buzzing. Nat yelled for me.

"Yo," he said, "you aren't gonna give up on the band, right?"

"Why would you even ask me that?"

"And we are never—*ever*—going to get lame-ass desk jobs, right?"

I laughed. "I couldn't even imagine."

"Good," he said, "me either. All right, Jason, go for it."

Before I grasped what was happening, Jason dug the needles into my brother's neck.

* * *

Nat and I didn't get home until three in the morning. The lights of the house were out, except the glow of the TV from the living room.

I walked through the kitchen—a bottle of wine sat uncorked on the counter. The kitchen table was littered with papers and white envelopes. I squinted at them in the dark. Medical bills. Late notices. Insurance paperwork.

Mom was in the living room, asleep in the corner chair. A half-empty wineglass sat forgotten on the floor. The TV played an infomercial.

"Mom," I said, shaking her gently.

Her eyes flickered open. She looked at me, confused. I couldn't tell if she was drunk or dreaming. She rubbed her hand over her face.

"It's late," I said. "You should go crash out."

She nodded and stood up. Her eyes locked onto the Saran Wrap covering my left arm.

All of a sudden, she looked very awake.

She grabbed my arm. I jerked back in pain.

"*Shit!*" I cried. "Chill out."

"My God, Rob. You're smarter than this!" she said, disgusted.

"It isn't a big deal."

She started to reply but stopped—she'd spotted Nat behind me.

"I hope *you're* happy now," she said to him.

Nat ignored her completely. He opened the door to the basement.

Mom's eyes grew wider than wide.

The light above stairs centered a perfect spotlight on the three big nautical stars that now ran permanently down the side of his neck.

"*WHAT DID YOU DO!*" she yelled.

She rushed toward him. She grabbed his shoulder and pulled him toward her. She let out a deep, guttural noise and then pushed him away.

"*Aren't things bad enough in this house? Why are you doing this? Why?*"

The rest of her words were incoherent mumbling. She pushed past Nat, disappearing into the dark hall. I heard her stumble up the stairs, crying.

Nat shook his head. "Mom is losing her fucking grip, man."

We were *all* losing our grip, but no one had let go yet.

Nat shut the basement door behind him. I let out a long, hopeless sigh.

2

A blue envelope arrived in the mail. It was addressed to me. Inside was a check from the Social Security Office for $733.31.

I asked Dad about it when he got home from work.

"It's for disability," he said. "You can cash it—it's your money."

"I don't need disability, man."

"Yes," he said. "Yes, you do. That's why I signed you up."

"What the hell?"

"I had to. Your mother's insurance company is trying to deny some of our recent claims."

"Why would they do that?" I asked.

He shook his head. "Because it's a cold goddamn world, big boy. But it will all be fine. This is just a way to prove that you are, in fact, disabled now. Which means you'll stay covered until we get this stuff sorted out."

More new shitty things.

"We got a letter saying that—officially—under your mother's current plan, the definition of a 'respiratory disability' has been changed from having less than forty-six percent breathing capacity to having less than *forty* percent breathing capacity—like they just happened to change her plan the week after we turned in paperwork stating your capacity is up to forty-five percent."

"*What the hell?* Can they do that?"

"Unfortunately," he said. "Insurance is one of the biggest rackets of them all."

"Is that why all those bills were lying out the other night?"

"Some of them. Only about two million bucks' worth," he said nonchalantly, and slapped my arm. "Don't let it rattle you."

*　*　*

A week later, I went to Columbus for a follow-up with Dr. Ranalli. Everyone at the hospital seemed excited to see me. Dr. Ranalli couldn't believe I'd had the balls to actually get the tattoo. Stacey petted my hair.

Dr. Ranalli said that he and Dr. Einhorn believed only two more rounds of chemo would be necessary. My blood work was looking good, my tests were looking good—two more rounds, and I'd be on my way to remission.

Stacey scheduled the first round for the second week of September. While she did paperwork, Mom told Dr. Ranalli about the issues with our health insurance.

I tried to tune it out. Thinking about all that money made me feel anxious and guilty and just plain sad.

Millions of dollars . . . millions of hours . . . millions of cells . . . millions of songs . . . millions of days . . .

Wasted. Stolen. Taken away from us, because of this fucking cancer. I couldn't think about this. I couldn't be here.

Without a word, I stood up and left the room.

I rushed through the waiting room, keeping my eyes forward and low. I needed to get out. I needed to move forward. The smells, the kids with the missing hair . . . missing limbs . . . deep-set, naked eyes . . . goddammit . . . I just needed to get *out*. . . .

TWENTY-TWO

The Blackest Black

1

Ali and I sat in the backyard with our feet in the kiddie pool. The water was lukewarm. The bright blue plastic was now a bleached-out, exhausted version of itself, a signal that the summer had finally run its course.

Ali looked tired. Or maybe stoned. Maybe both. I didn't ask these days. She gave me company, and that was enough. She came over a lot that week, the last before school started up again. The combination of the two of us, each on our separate drugs, made for some interestingly weird conversations.

"Do you think you'll go back to school at all?" she asked.

I shrugged and picked another layer of skin off my peeling tattoo.

"Will they let you graduate if you don't? Do you think they'd fail you if you're still too sick to go?"

"I won't be 'too sick,'" I said, "not for long. But I still might not go back. Fuck it, you know? I don't really care if they fail me or not."

Ali nodded. Her tan calves were above the water.

"I don't want to go back either," she said. "Not really, anyway."

"What do you wanna do instead?"

She thought it over.

"Be a lifeguard, maybe."

"Yeah? Can you swim? I've never seen you do anything at the pool except lie out and smoke cigarettes."

"Hey, that's bullshit!" she said, kicking water up at me. "Okay, okay, I don't, like, *swim*—but I wade."

"You wade?"

She nodded. "Yep. I wade."

"I'm not sure wading fits the job requirements."

"Oh, I know. I figured they'd hire me for my tits."

It was hard to argue with her logic.

We both zoned out and looked up at the cloudless sky. Our toes made ripples in the shallow pool as we spent our last summer days in our summer daze.

2

School was back in session. My parents were back at work.

I was back on the floor. I dozed through my afternoons to the soothing sounds of daytime TV trash. I hated it. I tried to exercise—but I couldn't. I was too weak. I was in too much pain. So mostly, I slept.

By the second week, it got to be too much. I didn't feel like sleeping—I was all slept out. I didn't want to lie on the goddamn floor. I didn't want to watch shitty TV.

What I wanted to do—what I *needed* to do—was play drums.

But this opened the door to problems reaching way beyond my breathing.

For one thing, I wasn't supposed to lift my arms higher than a tabletop. Whenever I did, the skin in my underarms stretched. Although the staples had been removed, the wound across my chest was still fresh. Too much strain on the skin could open it back up.

For another, the nerve damage in my hands and feet would make it nearly impossible to grip drumsticks. Plus, Mom would murder me if she heard me practicing drums already. . . .

But I had to do it.

I couldn't wait any longer. All I had *was* the band, and if I was going to get us back where we belonged, I was going to have to start playing.

I tried to think of my body as a new body—one learning a skill from scratch. That meant starting slow, easing my way back into the groove.

I decided to start with the core elements—snare, kick, cymbal—just enough to get my limbs comfortable coordinating again. I would start with the same standard two/four beat that I'd learned to master when we first took to the basement.

I needed to practice in secret—no one could know that I was playing again, not until I got an official okay from the doc. Privacy meant avoiding the practice space. If the band claimed the underground, I needed to go higher.

I decided on Nat's old bedroom. He never used it anymore; he always slept in the basement. There were two locks on the door. It was perfect.

It took all day to move the equipment I needed upstairs from the basement.

I put a plastic warm-up pad on a snare stand. It had the same bounce as a real snare drum, but none of the noise or kickback. I brought my kick-drum pedal up, but I didn't bring the drum—it was too heavy to carry. So I just duct-taped the pedal onto the floor and taped a pillow to the wall in front of it for impact—now I could practice technique without a lot of noise. There wasn't much I could do to silence my cymbals, so I taped dish towels around them. Now they sounded like cracked wind chimes.

After I got my practice kit set up, I did a run-through.

When I hit the practice pad, my left stick flew from my hands. *Shit.* I wrapped the bottoms of my drumsticks with duct tape. I twisted it so the sticky side was still facing my palms.

I picked up the stick again. I felt it connect to my palm.

I hit the pad again. This time, it stayed under my control. I hit it again.

Even that small amount of movement winded me. I hunched over on my stool, aching horribly. But I heard real drums in my head as I banged on the makeshift practice set. I heard a full kit, echoing loudly off the walls of my brain.

And so I kept at it.

*　*　*

The school sent Nat home with stacks of homework for me—this year, I was expected to work at the same pace as everyone else. Calculus, Spanish II, Bio II, Health—I tossed it all onto a pile of old magazines and I never looked at it again.

I didn't have time for that useless bullshit. In a few weeks I would be sent back to Columbus. While I was home, I needed to focus on drumming, not on calculus problems that didn't affect me at all.

I could only stand to practice for about five minutes at a time. My back and chest hurt badly, and my duct-taped drumsticks tore at the skin of my fingers. I hit the drums lightly, a far cry from how I used to pound on them—but no matter how gently I played, every downstroke made me wince in pain.

I worked in small, frequent intervals, the same way I had exercised before the surgery. I tried to practice five times an hour. That meant no more sleeping in, no more TV bingeing—as soon as everyone was out of the house, I got out of bed and went to work.

As hard and painful as playing was, the feeling I got afterward (*progress!*) outweighed the hurt. I'd worked up from a two/four beat to a four/four beat and was slowly relearning my snare rolls. I started to work on accenting a backbeat—the note that sits *behind* the notes, nudging them along, making them groove, filling songs with energy and sex, and making music worth listening to.

Beat by beat, I felt myself coming along. I drummed slowly, painfully, and ceaselessly. I played through the hurt.

It was with that same mind-set that I stubbornly forced myself to exercise again. The pain was horrible, but I knew I wouldn't make any serious strides drumming until I could build my strength back up. Doing just five or six push-ups was excruciating, and left me breathless to the point of panic.

But I reminded myself that I'd be in pain either way, so I might as well get something done. If I expected to bend my own destiny, it was time I started pushing.

3

The night before I posed for what would be our last band photos, I dyed my growing-in hair jet-black. Eyebrows too; I colored it all the blackest black I could—Halloween black, *Danzig* black, that unnatural shade of dark that only comes in a bottle. The same bottle my brother used.

My bangs had grown almost half an inch long, which was nothing short of a miracle. It was still thin in certain patches, but at least it was mostly there. The dye sharpened the arches of my eyebrows, making my eyes glow blue and alive.

I used Dad's shoe polish to fill in the spots where my hair was thin—fuck it, it looked believable enough.

I stared at myself in the mirror for a long time. When I took off my glasses, I looked more like my brother than I had since we were little kids—for once we actually looked *identical*. . . .

But really, we weren't identical at all. He was this grown-up now, moving along on a different path. And I was becoming this new thing, fragile in places, harder in others.

I found that I was beginning to get used to the idea.

Nat was decked out in black everything. He wore leather shoes. He was braceleted, chained, tattooed, and pierced—he looked like rock 'n' roll personified (or at least too cool to be sitting in our living room).

"Is my outfit"—work pants, Social D T-shirt, *Fuck Cancer* Chucks—"all right?" I asked him.

He nodded. "You look legit." He tossed me a small tube of lotion. "Put some of that on your tattoo, man. Those colors will pop bright as shit."

I squeezed a gob of lotion out and rubbed it on my forearm—he was right; the clouds grew darker, the stars glowed with purpose. Nat straightened his arm next to mine, and the tattoos blended together as one.

"Admit it," he said. "We look good as fuck."

Brody came over in his standard wife beater and cabbie hat. The three of us were standing in front of a brick wall, in the alley behind our house. Paul said that if he cropped the photo tight, it would look like it'd been taken on a city street.

He directed the shoot—*Stand here. Okay, Nat, move up three inches. . . . Wait. Chin down, Brody*—and kept reminding us not to blink. He took the photos with a camera that he'd swiped from school.

It was a sunny day, and the glare from my glasses made it hard for me to keep my eyes open.

"The squinting looks fine," Paul told me, over the sound of shutter snaps. "It makes it look like you're scowling. Shit, it makes you guys almost look tough."

*   *   *

After Paul ran out of film, he considered the shoot a wrap. The four of us walked down the alley, toward the front of the house. As we hit the front sidewalk, I saw Doyle leaning against his car. He was parked right in front of Sheena. He waved, smiled.

Nat looked as confused as I was. Doyle put his hands in his pockets and walked toward us.

"Hey y'all," he said.

"Uh, what's up?" Nat asked.

Doyle shrugged. "Brody called and said y'all needed me to come by."

Nat looked at Brody. "Well? So what's up?"

Brody cleared his throat. "I figured, you know, while we're taking new band pictures we might as well, like, take some with Doyle in them."

"Why?" I snapped.

Doyle looked between the three of us nervously.

"Why? Why do you think?" Brody said. He spoke louder now. "Do you even know how many people saw us at those Warped Tour shows, dude? *Thousands*—thousands of people, who would recognize Doyle as Defiance of Authority's drummer. I mean, what if someone—someone important—had seen our set and loved us, but never caught the band name? If they see a band photo and recognize Doyle, then it would jog their memory. Shit! It could land us a record deal—you never know."

"Warped Tour is *over*," Nat said. "Rob's still the drummer of this band."

Doyle put his hands up. "Hey, I didn't know this is why I was supposed to come by. I think it's somethin' you boys need to sort out yourselves. I'm gonna split."

304

"No," Brody said. "Hold up a minute, Doyle. This fucking concerns you too. Rob, we've decided that—*for the good of the band*—we need to start playing shows again. I know that keeping Doyle in the band bums you out, but if we wait any longer we'll lose all the momentum and exposure we got."

"We?" Nat said. "What the hell are you talking about? I've never said *anything* like that—*ever*."

"Me either, dude," Doyle swore.

Brody huffed. "Okay—not *we*, apparently—*me*. Is that better? And yes, I know Doyle was just supposed to join up for that tour—*but plans have obviously fucking changed!* If you don't agree, then you're kidding yourselves. I mean, you can barely make it up a flight of stairs, Rob! How are you going to play drums? It isn't going to happen, dude—you need to accept it."

"Bullshit," I mumbled. "That's fucking bullshit."

"He'll be able to play again," Paul said.

"Yeah. Okay. That positive-outlook crap is great and all—but you need to understand that if you *do* get to the point that you can play again, you'll have already screwed me, Doyle, and *your own brother* out of a music career." He turned to Nat. "You keep talking about these new songs you're supposedly writing—don't you think I already have plans to get them out? Don't you think I'm already brainstorming on our next move? *We can't just wait around!* If we do, everyone will forget us. We'll be yesterday's headlines and we'll have to start from zero, and I refuse to do that. I *refuse.*"

"Jesus! Just shut the fuck up," Paul yelled. "Do you realize how horrible you sound right now?"

I watched Nat's fists clench and unclench.

"Rob only has two more chemotherapies left," he said slowly. "We are waiting to play *any* shows, to record *any* songs, until he is ready to roll. Period."

"Yeah," Doyle said, backing toward his car. "I don't really feel cool with this, Brody. I mean . . . damn." He shook his head.

Brody threw up his hands. He stormed over to his Jeep.

"You really want to shoot our band—*your* songs—in the foot, don't you Nat?" he said, as he opened the door. "You better think this shit over—because I've worked too fucking hard to just let you guys blow this."

Brody slammed his car door. I didn't know what to say. I was sweating. I ran my hand through my hair. Streaks of black shoe polish covered my palm.

TWENTY-THREE

Symptoms of Me

1

On the cancer ward, life doesn't change.

The patients are indistinguishable, a collection of hairless lab rats whose owners struggle to tell them apart. The drugs go in, the life goes out. Time is only measured with befores and afters.

But this time, I felt like an outsider.

I didn't feel sick anymore. I didn't feel good, exactly, but I *didn't feel sick*. My hair had grown back. My face looked like *me* again. My new body was scarred and tattooed, and my muscles brimmed with tension and life. I felt like I was regaining control of myself.

When they injected the first bag of my chemo cocktail, I tasted familiar chemicals.

But now, I wanted control.

Stubborn, pointless control, any that I could hold on to at all.

I refused to eat all day. I wouldn't sleep at night. I sat straight-backed in my chair, just like I had before, ignoring any thoughts or sensations.

I wouldn't speak. I was afraid that if I opened my mouth I would puke. Most of my communicating was done through annoyed nods—most of them meaning NO.

NO, I don't want to lie down. *NO* lights. *NO*, I don't want to talk/walk/eat/move.

YES, leave me alone.

I pursed my lips. I shut my eyes. The taste inside my mouth grew strong enough to smell. I'd forgotten how horrible this first dose of chemo could be. Thoughts bubbled up, breaking my concentration—images of recent meals: grade-D hamburger covered in melted Frosty, Big Gulps spilling over with cold pizza grease, chewed lettuce, refried beans, histories of compost now oozing together beneath radioactive microwaved rays.

Mom asked me if I was okay. I nodded curtly—*YES*.

Then I hacked gallons of green and pink toxic pukeshit all over my lap, feet, chair, trash can, floor, bed, and mom.

One day in, and I didn't feel so new or strong anymore.

*   *   *

The treatments made me sicker than they ever had, even back in those first days at Columbus Children's. I was too sick to take my pills—I puked them up before my stomach could process them into my bloodstream. With each hack and gag, the wounds from my surgery felt as if they were reopening, and the bed made my back hurt worse than ever. I tried to take my painkillers, but they wouldn't stay down.

Two days into my treatment, Dr. Ranalli began to

question his decision to restart the chemo so soon. He saw my severe reaction to the drugs, and worried that my body wasn't as far along in the healing process as they had hoped.

But I assured him that I could take it. As much as I couldn't stand the treatment, it wasn't as bad as prolonging things even further. I told Dr. Ranalli that I was strong enough to tough it out.

I'm not sure that anyone was buying it. The chemo was already starting to break me down.

Sometime during the third day, I noticed hair on my blanket and hospital gown. I ran my hand over my head—more thin black hairs stuck to my fingers and palm. I blew on my hand and they wisped away.

I wanted to weep.

On the morning of the fourth day, noises woke me.

"Turnthatfuckin' TV off," I croaked.

My throat was dry from sleep. The shades were drawn; powerful rays of sunlight squeezed through the edges, but around me the room was still dark. I squinted and called out. No one answered me.

Morning was a confusing time—ever since my return to the hospital, I hadn't been able to sleep without sedation. So at first, I thought maybe I was dreaming.

I groaned again and reached for my glasses. Mom came into focus. She stood at the edge of my bed. She was staring at the TV.

The *Today* show was on, but it didn't seem like the real *Today* show. Off camera, people were screaming. Smoke was everywhere. There was no way that I was looking at the same bright morning.

Then, everywhere, everyone was screaming. A building was burning. A building was falling.

The world was ending. It was all just a dream.

2

That entire day was confusing. I tried to focus on the television. I asked Mom questions, which she had no clue how to answer. The more news that came across the screen, the more confused I got.

For the first time ever, all the TVs in the cancer ward were on, blaring together as one depressing chorus. Kids got their treatments while parents and visitors stood glued to the screens at the feet of their beds. The more thoughtful parents huddled around the portable TV at the nurses' station.

The hospital staff—to their credit—was acting pretty normal. No one wanted to scare a building full of sick kids more than they already were. Nat ditched school and drove up as soon as the towers fell. He arrived sometime in the evening, before I'd finished my dose. He didn't interrupt me, but I could hear him bickering (as was the new normal) with Mom in the hallway.

A nurse came in to check my IV. The last bag was almost empty.

"I'd ask if you're okay," she said, "but it seems a silly question on such a horrible day."

She didn't expect a response. She emptied my trash can and set it beside me. She shut the door gently and left me alone.

*   *   *

The strange week dragged on.

The three of us watched TV every morning. Speeches and threats were given as facts and speculations slowly emerged. Rescue workers toiled in rubble. Photos of the missing covered chain-link fences.

The morning news was my window. The world beyond looked like one big unmarked grave.

While I got chemo during the day, Nat roamed around Columbus alone. The attack had shaken something in him, even if he was too much of a rock star now to admit it.

In the evenings, he always found his way back to the hospital. He and Mom greeted each other wordlessly; she was angry that he'd ditched school, she was angry about his neck tattoo, she was just *angry* with him, period. But they remained cordial as long as they were around me.

I still felt horrible, but for once I accepted I had no right to bitch. The nausea, the nerve damage, and the pain paled in comparison to what was happening outside my hospital walls.

So I tried not to whine about my back. I tried not to lash out when I was at my lowest. I tried not to get depressed about the black hairs I kept finding on my pillow and blanket and shoulders.

I tried to be tough—or, more accurately, I tried to only be a pussy on my own time.

*   *   *

Dr. Ranalli delivered my discharge papers himself. The cancer markers in my blood were the lowest they'd ever been, which he said was amazing. My hearing was worse by another seven percent. My breathing, by his new numbers, was down as well—to forty percent capacity, the exact cutoff number listed in our new insurance mandate.

"I sent a copy of *these* results, along with a personal letter, to your insurance agency earlier today," he told Mom. "Hopefully now you have one less thing to worry about."

Mom jumped up and hugged him. I gave a relieved smile—I was happy to give up my pulmonary numbers if it meant an end to our battles with the insurance company. What's a couple of short breaths versus millions of dollars?

Dr. Ranalli prescribed me a breathing steroid, which he hoped would help my lung function. Once I could stomach taking pills again, I needed to add it to my daily regimen. I smiled at this news too, imagining how a steroid might help with my workout routine.

Dr. Ranalli nodded at Nat's neck tattoo.

"At least you won't get drafted with that thing," he said.

"No way," Mom said. "He isn't going to get off *that* easy."

I told Mom that she could go ahead and leave, and that I would just catch a ride home with Nat. She looked slightly hurt but didn't protest. She hugged us both and left, promising to get my prescriptions filled on her way home.

I changed into my people clothes. Black hairs fell around me as I pulled the neck of my T-shirt over my head. I avoided the mirror.

I got nauseous as soon as we pulled into German Village traffic. I yelled for Nat to pull over, but we were stuck at a light. I opened the car door and barfed all over the BMW beside us. The light turned green and Nat sped off, laughing.

Once we got out of the city, I felt better. The afternoon sunlight was almost gone, save for a thin orange sliver stretching over the fields like a crack in a door. We drove past one of the farmers' markets that lay in the empty nowhere between Circleville and Chillicothe.

One by one, we passed hand-painted road signs advertising pumpkins, raisin pie, and homemade fudge. But the last signs of the row were different—they had been painted in a hurry, and their words were smeared and uneven. Nat read them out loud as we passed. . . .

UNITED WE STAND!

GOD BLESS AMERICA!

SUPPORT R PREZ!

"That's kinda nice," I said. Nat laughed again.

"*Shiiiiiiiiit,*" he said, "it's scary is what it is. Welcome to the new world order, man. Just you wait and see."

3

Those first days home, I didn't venture farther from my bed than the bathroom. I puked and slept as the post-terror world took shape.

New York became a beacon of brotherly love and combined sacrifice. Memorials and fund-raisers were held all over the world. The Who even got back together. America had taken one collective breath and sent millions of prayers out into the ether to accompany all the lost souls toward their respective gods.

But in our small town beside that big river, it was definitely not the dawning of the Age of Aquarius. As the days went on, and I became well enough to leave my house, I could sense a new paranoia spreading over Huntington.

I don't think that anyone was actually worried terrorists might crash a plane into the flea market or anything—the attacks that our citizens fretted over were more *symbolic*; not an attack on American soil, but an attack on "American values." This meant that anything, or anyone, considered outside the norm was suspect—including punks.

My first week home, Doyle was expelled from Ashland High because he wore an all-black outfit to school. His algebra teacher told the principal she was afraid he was part of the Trench Coat Mafia. Police even escorted him from school property.

A few days later, police arrived at *my* house. Paul and I were drinking iced tea on the front porch when two cruisers pulled up on the curb. They walked up the yard with their hands on their service revolvers. They questioned us for twenty minutes before they said that two of my neighbors had called them—they'd reported that Nazi skinheads were dealing drugs off my front porch. I told them that I had cancer, but I think they thought I was bullshitting.

The week after, Nat told me that YWCA management announced that, for the time being, they wouldn't be renting their hall for any political meetings, rock concerts, or other possibly subversive events. So, basically—no more shows.

The tie between teenagers playing music and terrorism was never fully addressed.

* * *

With all concerts canceled and nothing to do, the one bright side I saw was the chance to see more of my brother at home, but unfortunately, it wasn't the case.

I knew that things were tense between him and Mom, so I wasn't shocked that he spent a lot of time away. But I started to feel like he was blowing me off too—I worried it was because of that argument with Brody, the one on the day of the photo shoot, but I hadn't had the balls to bring it up to him yet.

Nat seemed to spend all his time with girls. Not Ashley, or anyone whom I even knew; random girls, who seemed to come out of nowhere. He said he'd met them all through the band. Who knows, maybe they'd been coming around for a while now and I simply hadn't noticed.

He always made them wait outside.

Jessica, Tristan, Jenny, Heather, I can't remember all their names. I watched them from the porch, listening to their shoes crunch over red and gold leaves as they rushed up the yard to meet my twin.

All the girls were prettier than Ashley, but none of the girls would talk to me. I was lucky if they even said hi.

At least Ashley is quiet because she's shy, I thought to myself, *not because she's a bitch.*

Paul was convinced that the girls copped attitude because they were jealous—as long as Nat had a sick brother around, they would never be his number one priority.

I told Paul he was crazy. Shit, those chicks probably didn't even know we were brothers—by that second week home, we already looked like strangers again.

That breathing steroid Dr. Ranalli prescribed had the opposite results of what I'd hoped for. I couldn't breathe any better, and I didn't feel stronger—I just felt antsy. Worse—the steroid made me gain an insane amount of weight, in an incredibly short amount of time.

I couldn't believe it—I was fat again.

Not even in my most pessimistic fantasies could I have imagined that I'd be a fat cancer patient. And not just fat. I was *puffy*. The medication made my entire body swell up; I looked like I'd walked into a hornets' nest.

The last of my dyed-black hair had blown away. Even my eyebrows were gone. The more I puffed up, the fewer defining features remained. I was just a white, hairless glob of shit. I was an ugly marshmallow. I stood in the bathroom, cursing my puffed cheeks and fat neck, disgusted by the way my bloated crotch overtook the most impotent cock in teenage history. My scar looked pathetic now; my tits flopped lazily over it, their nipples pink and swollen.

Every single day, mirrors broke my heart.

And my brother, with his girls. That was a different kind of mirror—reflecting his high, thick hair and his healthy body, highlighting the newfound confidence on his almost handsome face. Every time I looked at him, or saw his arm around a girl, I felt like I was peering at an image of myself—that could have been. That might have been. That was not.

4

"Why the hell would you even *ask* me about college?"

I was lying on the floor of my bedroom with the phone receiver perched on my stomach. I twisted the cord around my fingers, annoyed.

"I don't know," Ali said. "It's coming up soon, is all. Tyson and Jamie already got into OU, and all my friends are done sending out applications. I just figured, like, maybe we should too."

"*We*—uh-huh, right. You mean *you* should."

I could hear her sigh over the line. "I meant both of us, Rob. I don't know why you have to be like this."

"You don't? Really? Because for a minute, I thought maybe you were sober enough to understand that I have *way* too much shit going on to care about college applications!"

I covered the receiver so she couldn't tell I was out of breath.

"You don't have to be a dick about it. I just thought it might be something you would want to start planning for."

"My only plan . . . is no plans," I snapped. "*When I am in remission*, I'll make plans. But right now it's a waste of time. If you want to start applying and try to make a break for it, go ahead. I can't blame you."

"Of course I want to go to college," she said. "God, how many nights did *you* use to encourage me to do it. Maybe I can stay here and go to Marshall if I get enough financial aid . . . but I couldn't go out of state, even if I wanted to. I'm not trying to run away from *anything*."

"I'm not a fucking idiot. Chemo mighta fried my brain, but I'm not fucking *stupid*—all you want to do is run away! Run to stupid football keggers with your friends. Run to those gross frat houses. Run to go—"

"Stop it!" Ali cried. "I can't take any more of this! I'm sorry, for *whatever* I did to make you so upset. I'm sorry that you feel so bad, but Jesus, you are turning into the most miserable person I've ever met. Whatever you think is twisting you up like this—listen to me, babe, you are doing it to yourself."

Whatever, I thought once we hung up. *Why the fuck would she ask me about college? Like I care. Mom and Dad don't even give a shit about it.*

Which was true—my parents never brought up college, not since the day I got sick. They humored my plans of becoming a rock star, like it was as reasonable and clear-cut as deciding to be a podiatrist.

They figured that my dreams gave me hope. What was the harm in them? They didn't want me to plan to enter school in the fall, because they knew there was a chance I might still be sick. They did my schoolwork for me and had me sign my name. They dealt with pretty much *everything* for me so I could focus on my rock 'n' roll fantasies.

It was easier on me—and them—if I continued dreaming up my own path, one with no plans, no viable future.

And, really, what could be more punk rock than that?

*   *   *

Nocomply11: I don't know. I think maybe I've spread her 2 thin. All her friends hate me, and I can't blame them, really. Lately whenever she parties with them I get on her case.

CynamnGirl84: why?

Nocomply11: I guess cause I am spread thin too? Frustrated. Just every time I look at her now, I see some kinda guilt—and it makes me feel worse. Like she has no reason 2 b guilty for just wanting to b normal. U know?

I was logging on to America Online a lot more. I didn't have anything else to do. I talked with Babs almost every day, sometimes in the CancerKidz chat, sometimes privately.

Talking with her helped my mood. It wasn't like talking to Nat or Ali, not that they had much time to talk lately, anyway. I could vent to Babs, and I could try to get ahold of my feelings for once. And she could listen openly, without the weight of context to soil her vision.

So we talked. Every day. Ali was at school, Mom was at work, Dad was gone, Nat was *gone*, and I was shut away in another room, staring at a screen and talking to an invisible girl.

CynamnGirl84: U don't have anything to feel guilty about, rob.

Nocomply11: Yeah rite! I know u can't see how fukt

everything is here—when I first got sick, everything was good, better even. But after my surgery, it all just got too heavy. Like I am the weight around everyone's neck. Everyone's fighting, or not speaking, everyone's always pissed.

CynamnGirl84: That isn't your fault. The anger and stuff is probably just a symptom of depression, or stress.

Nocomply11: Yeah, maybe. But the stress and depression are symptoms of me.

I typed blindly, without forethought or pause. Sometimes I revealed thoughts that I would never have considered out loud. I guess I couldn't really understand the way I felt, until I typed it out. But once I had, it could not be unwritten.

I couldn't unsay those words, and I couldn't unfeel those feelings. I couldn't just push it out of my mind. After I turned off the computer and walked away from those raw conversations, I found that I observed my natural world with a new, bleak clarity.

Everything felt smaller, tense and tight.

5

I decided to try and push through this funk, salvaging what was left of my time at home. Control what I could control. If I could get stronger, then I could play drums, and if I was playing drums, Nat would have a reason to come home.

I convinced myself that if I exercised, as soon as I got off the breathing steroid the pounds and puffiness would melt away, only to reveal the hard, chiseled body of a pale Greek god beneath (I knew that realistically the chances were slim, but it was all that I could do to get outta bed).

To further motivate myself to get off my ass, I decided to make a game of my workouts.

Dad's old record collection was tucked away beneath the mantel on our living room wall. His dusty turntable sat on top of the VCR. Every day, I took a new record off the shelf—this would be my official workout music of the day, meaning I wasn't allowed to stop exercising until the record ended. I could force myself to keep going, while having something to focus on other than how crappy I felt.

Most of the LPs were shit.

It's hard to do curls listening to Leo Sayer, and no Mary Chapin Carpenter record has *ever* inspired someone to fight for a few extra push-ups. But some of the albums, I had to admit, kinda fucking ruled.

It didn't matter what results these workouts actually produced—they became a necessity to me. Exercise felt more important than all my medications combined. It felt more useful than prayer.

I couldn't control my illness. I knew that by now. I couldn't diagnose, prescribe, or wish away my problems—but I alone could control my body.

Anyone seeing me then—hunched over in my living room with my parents' stereo cranked up to the max, gasping for breath while my trembling arms struggled to lift dumbbells to the blasting sounds of Springsteen or

CCR—likely would have been disturbed. But it was all I could do to feel like I was a participant in the fight for my life.

*　　*　　*

"Mom!" I screamed as I ran into my parents' bedroom.

It was six in the morning. The news was on. Mom was dressing for work. Dad was drinking coffee.

"What? What is it?" she asked, confused.

"My fucking arm!"

I held up my right arm—it was so swollen it wouldn't even bend at the elbow. Her eyes grew wider.

"Did you do anything to hurt it?"

I shook my head. My heart was racing.

"Have you overworked it?" she asked.

"I don't know, Mom. I don't think so. I just woke up and it was like this."

She sighed.

"Well, get dressed, honey. I need to call my office and tell them I can't come in. I have to take you back to the hospital."

It was a blood clot. Doctors and nurses had warned me about them, but I never really expected to get one.

The ER doctor was pretty freaked when he saw my arm. He started me on anticoagulation medications, and Mom got him in touch with Stacey at Columbus Children's. The drugs made my head throb.

The ER doctor came in after he'd spoken with Stacey. He told us that I needed to go to Columbus Children's

Hospital immediately, so they could scan for other clots and better monitor my treatment.

"Columbus," I said to Mom. "He's kidding, right? I still have a week before my next chemo—I don't wanna spend it there!" I looked at the doctor pleadingly. "Can't you just give me some of this medicine to take at home? I'm fine."

"Sorry," he said. "Blood clots can't be taken lightly—especially with a patient in your condition."

"It can't be that big of a deal," I said.

"Robert, let me make this clear—the clot in your veins could stop that heart of yours before the cancer even gets warmed up. You got me?"

I got him.

Mom and I rushed home to pack our bags.

*   *   *

Four days.

Another four fucking days I spent in the hospital. And not even on the cancer ward—I was stuck in some gen-pop room, beside a little kid in a body cast. They strapped leg massagers on me to circulate my blood, and the nurses only let me up to piss or get ultrasounds.

Otherwise, I was literally stuck in bed, wide-awake and frustrated as hell, listening to my cell mate moan incoherently through the curtain between us. I wondered if I had done this to myself—had I pushed my body too hard? Had I screwed up this bad, forced myself back into the damn hospital?

No one visited. No one called. Four days I lay there, thinking these thoughts, until they finally let me go. They sent us home with two new medications and five packs of heparin-filled syringes that I had to inject into my stomach once a day. I didn't really mind the pain anymore.

*　　*　　*

Back home, the distance among my family had spread. Dad went in to work earlier and stayed out later. Mom seemed perpetually stressed and overwhelmed. My brother didn't come home at all. The high school called, because he was never in class.

"Do you know what he has the house number saved as in his cell phone?" Mom asked one night at dinner. She was glaring at Nat's empty chair.

I sighed. "What?"

"Hell!" she said. "He thinks this is *hell*."

Her tone broke into words meant for only her ears.

"I *try* so hard to keep all this together," she mumbled. "God*, I am a terrible mother.*"

"Jesus, Terri," Dad said. He stood up from the table. He tossed his plate into the sink. Food scraps and silverware bounced off the counter. "You've *got* to get a grip!"

He stormed up the stairs. I heard their bedroom door slam. Mom sat at the table and cried.

Late that night, when my parents were in bed, I heard Nat coming in through the basement window. I found him down there, throwing clothes into a backpack.

"Yo, dude," I said.

He looked surprised to see me.

"Oh, hey. Didn't know you were back. How are you feeling?"

"All right. Totally dumb that they kept me in the hospital that long."

He nodded. "I was gonna come up and visit, but like every day Dad would say they were about to let you leave."

"No worries," I said, "it was all a clusterfuck."

He held out his arm. "Check *this* out, though."

He had a new tattoo—a bomb on his opposite forearm, with the words *Skate and Destroy* around it.

"Sweet," I said, trying to remember the last time I'd seen him on a skateboard. "When did you get that?"

"The other night. Jason hooked me up for pretty much nothin'."

I nodded at his backpack on the floor.

"Where are you going?"

"I've been crashing over at Jessica's . . . remember, the blonde? She has an apartment near the old post office."

"Are you dating her now?"

"I wouldn't say *dating*," he said.

"So Ashley split?"

He ignored the question and pulled the cushions off the love seat, grabbing the change beneath them. Then he continued packing his bag. He took a pair of Converse from the corner and stuffed them in last.

"When'd you get a pair of Chucks?"

"Ah" he mumbled, "actually, they're yours."

"Mine?"

"Yeah, well, you hadn't really been wearing them much lately. So I figured I could borrow them."

"Wait. You mean my *FUCK CANCER* shoes?"

"Yeah. I mean, I marked over the words in Wite-Out, so they didn't look as crazy."

"Why the hell would you do that, man?"

"Chill out," he said. "I didn't think you'd care. You're pretty much cured, right? I figured that's why you weren't wearing them. I didn't think it was a big deal."

I didn't know quite what to say. Neither did he. He stood there awkwardly for a moment, and then he moved past me without another word.

He propped himself up to the open window.

"Hey," I said behind him. "You maybe wanna go to the movies tomorrow or something?"

"Sorry, dude. I can't."

"Oh. Okay."

Nat tossed his bag out the window. He lifted himself with a grunt, struggling to wiggle through the tiny frame.

Before I walked upstairs, he ducked his head back inside.

"*Rob?*" he whispered. I walked over.

"Don't tell anyone where I'm at, okay? Don't tell Mom that I came by."

"Yeah, sure," I said. "I won't let anyone know."

"Thanks," he said.

Then he was gone.

I walked slowly up the stairs. I switched off the basement light. I caught my breath in the dark, then made my way to my bedroom. I kept the basement window open, in case my brother found the way back home.

TWENTY-FOUR

The Imprints of Angels

1

Mom got a phone call from her supervisor on the evening before we left for Columbus—due to the increased terror level, the federal government was imposing new security mandates for all oil refineries. A mandatory staff meeting was scheduled so they could work through the transitions and getting the refinery up to code. The meeting was to be held in two days.

It was one of life's little ironies, the way the timing worked out. My mom was called in to work, just as she had been on the day of my diagnosis. Now, for the first time since, it was my dad who needed to take me to the hospital.

I didn't get a chance to see my brother before I left. Not that I especially *needed* to see him, but it seemed important, nonetheless. I'd waited up for him on Sunday, but he never came home. I tried his cell—it was off. I didn't bother leaving a message.

Now, Dad and I traveled in silence. I couldn't help thinking back to that bad day, but I secretly feared men-

327

tioning it could jinx our entire trip. I stared out the window of the car, watching bare branches twitch like claws in a flip book. Dad turned the volume on the radio down.

"So, how's Natty doing?" he asked.

"Your guess is as good as mine. I barely see him lately."

Dad nodded. "This year has been really hard on him. He's trying his best to be a good brother to you."

"I know," I mumbled.

"And you aren't the easiest guy to be around sometimes."

"Yeah, yeah, I know that too. What about Mom? How is *she*?"

Dad sighed. "She's really trying to be strong—you know she's done a damn good job of staying strong for you. She just hasn't bounced back from your surgery the way you have. The world weighs heavier on some people, is all."

"I can tell."

"But she's trying. You know how your mother is. She doesn't like anyone to see her seem vulnerable, especially you."

"I know."

Dad stared straight out the windshield.

"Did you know that she's been going to counseling twice a week?"

"Really?" I asked. "Since when?"

"Since after your surgery. She goes to a support group sometimes too—down at the hospital."

"Damn."

"She's never mentioned it?"

"Not to me."

"Well—exactly my point. She doesn't want you to

know how much effort it takes her to deal with this shit. I think this week will give her a lot of closure, finishing treatment and all. We can move through it, just like we have been—we just gotta keep rolling forward."

I nodded and looked through the windshield too. The road ahead was wide open.

*   *   *

It was the first day of the last time.

I was anxious. Not about the chemotherapy. I felt anxious in a confused sort of way, like how a convict might be anxious when he learns his parole has finally been granted. I was afraid that the acknowledgment of finishing treatment—of *beating cancer*—could somehow open me up to seriously bad juju.

I could imagine the scene: doctors rushing into my room, telling me that there was a mistake, that I wasn't actually better, that the cancer had spread, and that I wasn't going anywhere.

So I decided to say goodbye quietly.

I dreamt my goodbyes, sending farewell thoughts to every nurse, every doctor, every tech, every orderly. Good-lucks went out to every stranger and patient. I summoned short, silent prayers for each person who passed through this cancer ward. I asked God to credit any remaining luck I had left toward the patients around me—I wouldn't need it anymore.

I woke up one morning to the sound of a trash bag getting stuffed into the wastebasket. The janitor was back. I hadn't seen him in months. I sat up in bed and watched as he struggled to get the bag around the rim.

"Hey, man," I said sleepily.

The janitor turned around, confused. It wasn't *my* janitor, after all—this was some young guy, pale, with cropped red hair. It was just another stranger.

"Sorry if I woke you," he said.

"What happened to the other guy?"

"Who?"

"Uh, the *other* guy, you know, the old janitor. The black dude."

The new janitor glanced around nervously, like he wasn't sure if company policy allowed interaction with the sick kids.

"I couldn't tell ya," he said. "I just started last week. I heard a few of the older guys were retiring, but I didn't meet most of 'em. Sorry."

"Black guy. Older," I continued. "He was in the army—in Germany."

The new janitor shrugged.

"Sorry," he said again. He took the used trash bag out into the hall.

"I wonder if he went back to Germany," I said to the empty room. I imagined him in Hamburg, beautifully out of place, walking the streets with a G-string girl under each arm. I had to smile. "Yeah, I bet he did. Fuck fucking yeah, he did."

It was the last thought I had before I drifted back to sleep.

*　*　*

Stacey and Dr. Ranalli said their goodbyes early, on the morning before my last injection. They were both disappointed that they weren't able to say goodbye to my mom too.

"This isn't *technically* goodbye," Stacey said, "which is good for me, because I'm selfish and I'll miss you! Ha-ha. But you'll only have to put up with me once a month now, when you come back to get your scans."

"I think I can handle that," I said.

She smiled and then turned to Dad. "Like we've discussed, from now on he'll be able to get his weekly blood work locally. They'll send the samples back here for examination. But he'll still need to come get his scans once a month."

Dad searched his pocket for a pen to write all of this down. Stacey touched his arm.

"Don't worry," she said. "I've already spoken to Terri about it on the phone."

Dad laughed. "Whew, good. She's been calling me twice a day for status reports."

"Well, tell her the status is his blood work looks great— this is one lucky dude!" Dr. Ranalli said, grinning.

The two of them came to my bed and hugged me gently, sidestepping the tubes and cords and machines. They lingered for only a moment, and then they were gone— off to save other kids, off to other kids who still needed saving.

I sat there calm, unusually content. I waited for the nurse to come and inject me with my last hit of poison. I shut my eyes and dreamed one final, silent goodbye.

2

"So how does it feel?" Dad asked.

We were on the outskirts of Wheelersburg—almost home. I squinted my eyes shut, trying to control my stomach. My head was still spinning from the drugs.

"I don't know," I said slowly. "It doesn't really feel like anything. *Anticlimactic*, I guess is the word."

Dad nodded. "I know what you mean. That's just *life*, son—all the mountains you climb, all these dreams you obsess over—once you achieve them, it always leaves you at a loss."

"I feel—"

"Numb to it all? Yeah, I get that. . . ."

"No," I snapped. "Fuck, I . . . I feel like I'm . . . gonna puke . . . fuck . . . ."

Dad pulled off to the side of the highway. He slammed on his brakes, engulfing the car in a cloud of road dust. I opened the door, unfastened my seat belt, leaned over, and barfed all over the shoulder.

When I was finished, I wiped off my lips and sat back in the seat. I looked to my left—Dad was gone. I hadn't noticed him get out of the car. For a minute, I almost panicked, but then I saw him, standing on the other side of the road, waving me over.

I stepped over the puke puddle and carefully made my way across the blacktop.

Dad stood in front of a used-car lot. The lot was empty except for six cars, a trailer, and a sign that read JJ'S CLASSIC AUTOS.

These cars *were* fucking classics—JJ wasn't kidding. Their bright paint jobs were dull now, transformed into colors only time can create. Their beauty floored me; I thought cars like this only existed in the movies.

"I had one just like her," Dad said. He nodded toward a long sedan with a blue/purple tint.

"What is it?"

He ran his hand across the hood. "A '66 Merc Comet. Mine was cream, though, beautiful. V-8 engine. Damn, I loved that car."

"It is really cool . . . but man, look at *that*! That is the car!" I said.

All of a sudden, I forgot about my nausea. My breath shortened as I walked toward it.

The car was a slice of apple pie. Red—not dull, but *bright* red, the color of hard candy. It had a black convertible top. The grille was capped with two fog lights, which glared at the road like omnipotent eyes. The two back tires were raised like those of a stock car, and the word AVENGER wrapped boldly around them. The trunk was blunt, like a sawed-off shotgun. Between the taillights, shiny metal letters spelled out:

M-U-S-T-A-N-G

"Wow, it's a ragtop too," Dad said. "Looks like a '67, maybe a '68."

"I've never seen anything this cool in my *life*, man!"

I looked at all that black leather inside. I checked the price that was written on the windshield—$5,200.

"How much you got saved up?" Dad asked, reading my mind.

"Not sure. A little—but not *this* much. I could start saving, though. You think they'd still have the car by the time I could get the money together?"

"It's junk," Dad scoffed. "If they're starting at five grand, she probably doesn't even run. This must be a piece-of-shit car."

"No, no, no," I said. "No way. This car is perfect."

Dad crossed his arms and stepped back, looking at me beside the Mustang.

"You really like it that much?"

"I do," I said. "It's rad as hell. It's straight outta a fucking Bruce Springsteen song."

3

I didn't get a big welcoming committee. But Nat was at home, and that was enough. He and Mom were sitting in the living room, watching TV together. Mom hugged me hello, and it seemed like the entire house let out a collective sigh.

It was done. It was over. We were safe.

Now I needed to rest.

Nat followed me into the kitchen. "Hey, man, I want to talk to you about something."

I shook my head. "Not right now. I feel like the walking dead, dude—I just want to sleep."

I turned away from him and dragged myself upstairs.

Nat opened the door to my bedroom without knocking.

"Sorry, I know you're tired, I just figured the sooner

we deal with this, the better. I didn't want to bring it up while you were in the hospital."

I groaned and swung my feet onto the carpet. Nat leaned on the wall across from me.

"Bring what up?"

"The band," he said. "We need to talk about the band."

"What about it?"

"You remember the shit that went down when we took the new press pics?"

"Of course I do," I said.

"Yeah—well, I haven't been able to get it out of my head. I've barely talked to Brody since then. I just can't stop thinking about it."

"So what?" I asked. "You want to tell me that y'all are gonna start doing shows without me? Now that I'm done with chemo, and you don't feel so guilty about it?"

"*Nononono,*" Nat said. "I wanted to talk to you about kicking *Brody* out."

"Seriously? I know that he was being a dick, but he kinda had a point. I mean, y'all already have a drummer on deck—you can play shows without *me*, but not without a bass player. It seems nuts to kick him out."

"Fuck that," Nat said. "This is *our* band—you know it, and I know it. If anyone is leaving, it's him. After that blowup, I can't even stand to be near him."

"Well, shit." I hadn't been expecting this. "Where do we find a new bassist?"

"I already got one on lockdown."

"*Who?*"

"Doyle."

"My fill-in drummer?" I asked, confused.

"Yep."

"He plays bass?"

"Fuck yeah he does—a little bit, at least. It's the *bass*, dude! How hard can it be?"

"Point taken."

"Brody's an idiot for obsessing over playing shows. We don't *need* to play local shows. I don't care if we ever play this town again. It's small-time bullshit. What we *need* to do is record an album—we could play a show at the Y every single day and no one outside the city limits would ever notice."

He sat down on the bed beside me.

"I say, let's scrap all the old material. I have tons of new songs waiting to be arranged. If you start working on your drumming soon, and Doyle practices his bass, I figure we can take the entire winter to work out the new stuff. Then, we can pick the best of them to record—not another demo—but a *real* album, in a *real* studio."

"Fuck yeah!" I said. I started getting stoked.

"We can go ahead and map out a tour for the summer, and start calling clubs sooner, not later. If we get our record done by the end of spring, we can send copies out to every magazine and website there is. We can get reviews, maybe even interviews—build a *buzz*, you know? People will come to the shows that way, and record labels might actually notice us."

I was sold.

"By the time June rolls around, we're gonna have a new band, new songs, a new record, and a new tour booked to promote the shit outta all of it. I think that the day after graduation, we just hit the fucking road—and this time, we don't come back without a record deal."

"Hell yes," I said loudly.

I was breathing harder, and my chest felt tight. I had to steady myself on the bed.

"What are we gonna tell Brody?" I asked. "He is going to *freak.*"

Nat shrugged. "I dunno. I don't care, honestly—I can't play music with him anymore. The second he gave up on you, I gave up on him."

We sat beside each other in silence.

"When do we start?"

"Whenever you feel ready," he said. "While you were in Columbus I spent the week demoing all of my new songs. It's just me and a guitar—I recorded it with the old Dictaphone we used to use. They don't sound great, but still. I thought maybe you could go ahead and start brainstorming arrangements while those chemo drugs run outta your system."

"Sounds good," I said.

Nat stood up and opened the door.

"Anyway, I just figured you'd wanna get the ball rolling. I put the demo tape in the other bedroom. You know, the one with all the drums in it. You sneaky fuck."

He laughed and walked into the hall.

*   *   *

I woke a few hours later, sick. I walked to the bathroom and puked as quietly as I could. I flushed, and stood above the sink until my breathing slowed. My stomach wouldn't quit rumbling. I took a few pills.

Until the meds kicked in, I would never be able to get to sleep. There was no point getting back in bed. So I walked across the hall, to the other bedroom.

Nat had placed his demo tape in the middle of my practice pad. How long had he known that all of this was up here? Probably the whole damn time.

My old Converse sat beside the drum stand. Nat had rewritten *FUCK CANCER* on the white rubber tips, even bigger than the original sentiment. I grinned and picked them up along with the tape before shutting off the light.

I put my headphones on and inserted them into the stereo jack. I flipped the tape to side A—I pressed rewind till it clicked. I cranked up the volume in advance.

I pressed play.

I closed my eyes.

This was my brother as I had never heard him. Without the accompaniment of a band, his punk sneer sounded softer, more vulnerable. It was jarring to listen to, but for that exact reason, it pulled me in.

The first song was called "Never Stop Fighting." It was balls-out fast, a punk rock fight song with a chanting chorus hook.

The second song, "No Tomorrow," was a little slower. It was a song about living for the moment while an uncertain future lies ahead. I could imagine it with drums pounding, pushing the music to be as heavy as the lyrics.

The next song was "Brothers Forever."

Then there was "H-Town Angels."

The one after that was called "Terminal."

It was unnerving, how raw they were. They were nihilistic, heartfelt, brutal. They were totally and completely *ours*.

Every song sounded like a revelation. All these things that he wouldn't—*couldn't*—say to me, my brother was saying to me now. He was telling me he loved me, in a language that he knew I'd understand.

4

The weather was getting colder. Stronger winds blew the few remaining leaves from their branches, and all the colorful yards of the neighborhood began to turn a dull gray. But as the temperature dropped, my own life finally began to thaw.

I still struggled physically. Many of the side effects I'd experienced lingered, some even longer than I could've imagined. But I was able to manage them decently enough.

I wrapped my drumsticks and even my fork in hockey tape to help the ruined nerves of my hands grip. I sang songs in my head to mute the ringing in my ears. The chemo brain slowly faded away, though I still had blank spots now and again.

The pain was the hardest thing. It was constant and unrelenting. I told myself that all my exercising helped, and maybe it did, but any amount of relief I felt was more likely coming from the five or six hydrocodone I popped daily.

But regardless of it all, I truly felt like I was getting better—mentally, emotionally, spiritually—I didn't cling to dark feelings anymore, and I no longer felt the grip of resentment and fear.

For the very first time, I felt like I had begun to heal.

A lot of my positive energy came from watching the burden of that year ease down off my family's back. It was like a curse was lifted from my house or something. It didn't happen overnight—but slowly, things went back to normal.

Better than normal, even.

Nat kicked Brody out of the band within a week of our decision. It wasn't the long, dramatic scene I'd expected; Nat simply threw his bass equipment out into the street and told him to come pick it up. Brody never argued or tried to work things out—I guess my brother's strategy made it clear there would be no reconciliation.

The vibe in the basement became warmer, the way it was before life had complicated the simple joys of rock 'n' roll.

Nat set up camp down there again—but this time, it was permanent. There were no more groupie girlfriends, there was no more running away. He and Mom finally called a truce—he went back to school, and she stopped arguing about his tattoos, or about his goals. In fact, she seemed to give up arguing altogether.

My mom had finally regained her focus. With me out of the hospital, she was devoting her free time to raising money for cancer research. She participated in charity walks and golf tournaments; she was even thinking of entering a marathon.

Her fund-raising helped her as much as it helped the

cause—she wasn't drinking much anymore, and now she stayed too busy to get depressed. She and Dad spent more time together—they even started going on dates. The color finally came back into her face, and I started hearing her sweet laugh for the first time in months.

When it was time to eat dinner, everyone showed up.

*   *   *

Ali.

I saw her less. I thought of her always. I thought of us ditching school. I thought of us dancing in the hospital. I thought of her watching me drum. I thought of our first kiss—but it was just so different now.

Every time I thought back to that kiss, I couldn't help but think of what came after. The heartaches, the fights, and the endless struggles—I couldn't separate the past from the present. I didn't know how to cherish those memories as singular experiences. The pleasure and the pain were all twisted up in my head with a sentimental clarity.

She wasn't a lover; she was a battlefield nurse. She wasn't a girlfriend; she was the weeping statue of Mary, crying rivers of tears for no one else but me.

She had transcended, in my mind and in my heart.

Ali Wilhelm was my very own saint.

I wish it could've been simpler, but I tried not to let it upset me. Mostly because I could tell that Ali was happier now.

When I came home from treatment that final time, she

was as relieved as anyone—relieved for me, and relieved for her. Because it meant she no longer had to feel guilty for yearning to *enjoy* her life.

Now she spent most of her time out with friends. They went to college parties and bars throughout the week, armed with stolen beer and ridiculous fake IDs.

Sometimes it made me worry—but what could I say? She'd stuck with me, through everything, and I owed her a lot for that. I felt like the least she deserved was some space.

So after all of it, I was once again nothing but a silent observer, a lonely boy just grateful to be in her presence.

* * *

It was just a few weeks before I started drumming for real.

I played the same simple beats on my real kit as I had on my practice set. But the volume and tone of actual drums brought those repetitive movements to life. The stick cracks and cymbal crashes rang in my head for hours—God, how I'd missed those sounds!

It wasn't much longer until I was jamming with Nat.

We played lots of old covers: Beach Boys, Misfits, Pennywise, the Descendents, Nirvana—any song we could remember. Getting back into the swing of it was exhausting, but that was fine—there was so much music, *sososo much awesome fucking music.*

Soon, we were hammering out the new material. We spent countless hours crafting arrangements, sculpting the songs from his demo into the most powerful shit we could. Doyle came by a few days a week, and he followed

Nat's chord changes on the beat-up bass he'd borrowed from a friend. He picked up the instrument relatively quickly, which wasn't a surprise—there was just something in the atmosphere around us now, and I knew that anything was possible.

I'd never enjoyed playing music so much. Practice never got stressful, and the songs never got old. We would stay down there all day, riffing and talking shit while Paul hunched in the corner, reading a magazine or snapping photos. When I was with my friends and my music, I finally felt like my struggles were over. When I was back behind my drum kit, I finally felt like I was home.

* * *

The afternoon before Thanksgiving, I walked into the kitchen to find Mom prepping her fruit salad. Her current project was raising money for the Ronald McDonald House. I asked her how it was going.

"Fast!" she said excitedly. "So far I've raised almost four thousand bucks. Pretty cool, huh?"

"Incredibly cool! That's so awesome. Seriously."

"You know," she said, "back in those first days, right when you were diagnosed, I felt so helpless. I remember sitting in that room with you, watching you sleep—so scared that I was going to do the wrong thing, make the wrong decision. Or not do *anything*, which seemed even worse." She smiled sadly. "I just kept telling myself that if we could get through it, I was going to do *something*. Help somehow. Anyway, I'm hoping that this money helps somebody. Not everyone is as lucky as us."

I envisioned her in the hospital, watching over my deathbed dreams. I didn't have the words to tell her what that meant, or how much she had done already. I knew, right then, that I never would.

So I simply nodded and looked away.

*   *   *

Whenever night came down and there was no more music to play, my brother and I focused on the road.

So far, Nat's plan was right on schedule. The songs were coming together nicely, and I couldn't have been more stoked to record them. I was sure that we were about to make a record worth listening to, a record someone like me would love. We still planned to track the album in early spring and have copies sent out for reviews by May.

Then, it would finally be time to tour.

Let me tell you, the first tour paled in comparison to the one we were lining up—we were gonna tour until we'd played every fucking city in the country, and then we were going to tour some more. We were going to tour until the wheels fell off.

Once again, Nat taped a map up onto the basement wall. This America had so many red stars drawn on it that it was hard to tell where the tour even began.

So far, we had fifteen confirmed bookings. We were sure we could lock in the rest of the gigs before the weather warmed up and club calendars got packed. Summer was the busy season, when every garage band in America got hungry for the promise of the road.

We planned to start on June 2, in Louisville, Kentucky. From there, we would go to Cincinnati to Indianapolis to Fort Wayne to Detroit to Chicago to St. Louis to Kansas City to Omaha to Sioux Falls to Fort Collins to Denver to Salt Lake City to Boise to Seattle to Olympia to Portland to Redding to Reno to San Fran to San Jose to Fresno to LA to Hollywood to San Diego to Vegas to Phoenix to Flagstaff to Albuquerque to Oklahoma City to Dallas to Houston to New Orleans to Birmingham to Memphis to Nashville to Atlanta to Jacksonville to Gainesville to Orlando to Miami to Tampa to Savannah to Charleston to Charlotte to Richmond to DC to Philly to New York to Asbury Park to Pittsburgh—and from there, to the triumphant homecoming gig in Huntington, West Virginia.

*   *   *

Every night before I went to bed, I took off my shirt and stood before the mirror. I needed to track the changes of my body.

Ever since I'd gotten finished with chemo and off the breathing steroid, my relentless workouts had begun finally showing some results. My arms and shoulders were bigger; the muscles in my chest bulged lopsidedly above my scar tissue.

My hair grew in slower this time, but I saw the shadow of progress on my head, jaw, and stomach.

I'd already blown all of my savings on tattoos. It had been less than two months, but my arms were nearly covered. And although it wasn't a conscious decision, each new tattoo was nothing but a remnant of that horrible year: a pinup nurse holding a needle, a death skull with my brother's words—*Never Stop Fighting*—surrounding it, the stained-glass mural from the Children's chapel, a daisy with a banner reading *MOM* in blue.

All of those experiences, relived in thick bright lines up and down my arms—as colorful as fantasies, but as permanent as a scar.

5

Blood work was on Tuesday afternoons.

I sat in the waiting room with the others; grayhairs bundled in layers of unmatched clothes, coughing and sniffling, barely awake. We waited for our names to be called.

My brother was with me that particular Tuesday, off school for Christmas break and bored with being at the house. He kept glancing at a patient in the far corner. She looked like a skeleton rotting inside an overcoat.

"This place is a fucking mortuary," he whispered.

I nodded—*yes, I know*.

A nurse with a clipboard came into the waiting room. She called my name.

I sat in a plush plastic chair and put my arm onto the armrest, the same type they used in the tattoo shop. The nurse didn't make conversation. She quietly tied off my arm—the veins bulging thicker now, because of the muscle—and stuck the needle in deep.

Every week they sent eight vials of my blood to Columbus. The results always came back clean. Those anxieties were behind me now—I was healed. The blood tests were just another mundane chore on my calendar.

After my arm was slapped with a Band-Aid, Nat and I made our way to the parking lot. It was snowing. I looked at the white sky and stuck out my tongue.

Snowflakes dissolved on my glasses. The van was totally covered. Nat cleaned off the windshield, stopping every few seconds to shake the snow from his hair.

By the time we got home, snow dusted every rooftop and branch. Snow painted all the yards and the street. It showed no sign of letting up.

Inside, I watched it fall through my bedroom window and tried to measure its height. Eight inches? A foot? It just kept pouring in a quick, slanted rush. Nat came to the window beside me.

"You know what this means?" he said. "Gobbler's Knob."

Gobbler's Knob—the most choice sledding spot in Huntington. It was behind the park, where the woods opened onto a clearing that just happened to be a steep-ass hill about three blocks long.

During the blizzard of '93, Nat and I had spent *weeks* there, flying down the Knob at bone-crushing speeds, oblivious to danger or death.

But our town hadn't had a good snow since.

"If it keeps coming down like this, that place will be *packed* tomorrow," I said. "Every brat in town will be there, hogging the whole hill."

"Exactly," he said. "That's why we should go tonight."

Nat called Paul about rustling up some sleds. I decided to call and invite Ali. I was surprised when she actually picked up the phone.

"Are you seeing this snow?" I asked.

"Yeah! I love it. The winters are usually so gray."

"Me and Nat are going sledding at Gobbler's Knob tonight. I wondered if you might wanna come."

"Tonight?" she said tentatively. "Okay, sure. But if I wreck the car driving down my hill I'm blaming you guys."

"I'll take the risk," I said. "At this point I'd say that we're goddamn untouchable."

*   *   *

I was bundled in three hoodies, a jean jacket, snow pants, a beanie, gloves, and an old pair of Docs. I felt like a tattooed penguin waddling to the van. The night air was freezing and felt sharp in my remaining lung. I began to worry about my breath but decided that there was no point—if Ali was going, I was going.

The storm left the neighborhood covered in the glow that comes with the snowfall dark. The night was bottom-lit, as if natural law had reversed itself. Nat drove slowly, careful to stay within the tire tracks of those before him. Paul waited on the sidewalk in front of his apartment. Three huge black inner tubes were stacked beside him. We slid to a stop.

Paul threw the tubes in the back of the van. He rubbed his hands together, shivering.

"Damn, what took y'all so long? I almost froze to death."

"*Sooooo* sorry, sweetheart." Nat laughed. "But these roads are complete shit. But hey, the inner tubes look perfect, man!"

"The tire shop on Second Avenue gave 'em to me for five bucks each. These mammas are gonna *fly*."

We pulled into the roundabout that marked the top of the Knob. Ali was already there, sitting in her car with her window cracked, smoking a cigarette. There were no other cars in sight. We parked beside her and walked into the cold.

"I almost skidded off the side of the hill," Ali said.

"But you *didn't*." I smiled, trying not to slip on the frozen ground.

She rolled her eyes and hugged me hello. She kissed me on the cheek. Her lips were warm.

"Fucking chick drivers," Paul said.

Ali punched him in his winter coat. We unloaded the inner tubes and headed toward the edge of the hill. I was really struggling, sucking frozen air in shallow puffs like a locomotive that's run out of coal.

The four of us peered over the edge.

The snow below was untouched, making the incline of the ground impossible to gauge. It was a blind drop.

We sat our tubes down in a straight row. We stood behind them, looking down, hesitating.

Paul's words were visible in the air—"Okay, pussies, do you want to live forever or something? Let's *go*!"

He took a running start and jumped face-first onto his tube, propelling it over the drop and out of sight.

We could hear him yelling.

Nat laughed nervously. He sat down in the middle of his inner tube like it was a pool float. He used his hands to drop over the edge.

He disappeared.

Ali and I held on to the sides of the last remaining tube. We pushed it forward, launching our bodies clumsily on board as the ground dropped out from under us.

She grabbed my jacket. We started to fall.

Snow blew around us like we were on the verge of an avalanche. It was hard to see. The tube twisted off course, spinning in uncontrollable circles like a hellish carnival ride.

We spun right. I saw Nat go flying off his tube.

"Wooooohhhooooo!" Ali cried.

We started to spin forward again and then crashed straight into Paul.

I was lying on my back.

My chest heaved. I heard laughter all around. I wiped the snow from my glasses and began laughing too—it made it even harder to breathe, but I just couldn't help it.

"Let's go again," Nat said from the ground across from me.

No one stood up. Soon, the laughter faded.

The four of us just lay there, silently breathing in the cold. The stars above us were tinted blue, like ice crystals frozen in heaven. The earth below them lay still. Our bodies cast the imprints of angels in the snow, but we were only kids.

TWENTY-FIVE

Out of Tune

1

Mom called to me from the kitchen. I switched the TV on mute.

"Dr. Ranalli is on the phone," she said. "He wants to know if you mind rescheduling your appointment next month, from January eleventh to January sixteenth."

I shrugged. "Yeah, whenever."

"I think he wants to talk to you."

Weird, I thought. *No doc has called me at home before.*

Mom handed me the phone.

"Hello?"

"Hey, Rob, Mark Ranalli here—how was your New Year's?"

"Okay, I guess."

"Great! I'm just calling to see if you can come in on the sixteenth instead of the eleventh."

"Yeah, Mom just told me. That works."

"Excellent," he said. "Oh, side note—didn't you once tell me that one of your favorite bands is Pennywise?"

"Yeah, why?"

"It just so happens that they're playing at the Newport

351

Music Hall in Columbus on the sixteenth, the day we just rescheduled your appointment."

"Really?"

"Also interesting—I happen to have a buddy who runs the Newport, and he happened to get me in touch with Pennywise's manager today. So you might ask your brother to drive you to that appointment—no offense to Mom—because there will be two VIP passes waiting at the box office. And just so you know, their manager said the band wants to meet you."

Meet ME?

"Are you fucking serious?" I said without thinking. He laughed into the phone.

"Think of it as a parting gift," he said, "from one old punk to another."

2

It was the morning of the sixteenth.

The van was crammed, and everyone was grumpy. None of my friends were used to being awake so early. Nat and I sat up front, listening to Pennywise CDs on repeat. Doyle, Tyson, and Paul took the bench seats. Ali slept in the back.

In my pocket was a copy of our old demo—the new songs we'd been working on were better, but until we had them recorded this would have to do. If I got the chance, I was determined to give the demo to the band.

By nine, the gang was walking me through the halls of Columbus Children's Hospital, earning odd looks from the families and staff. It was awesome to feel out of place inside these walls.

Before I checked in, I asked my friends to wait outside the oncology clinic—the waiting-room vibe usually rested somewhere between bleak and heartbreaking, and I didn't want the presence of my weirdo buddies making these cancer kidz even more uncomfortable. I told them I'd call Nat's cell when I finished, and they left to look for some trouble.

Pulmonologist. Audiologist. Cardiologist. PET scan. EKG. Normally all these appointments left me exhausted. But not today—today, I was buzzing.

After the EKG, a nurse showed me into an exam room to meet with Dr. Ranalli. But when the door finally opened, Stacey walked in alone.

"Mark was held up," she said. "It was an emergency. He wanted me to come tell you to get outta here—and to have a *great* time at the concert! We want a full recap."

"For sure," I said, jumping off the exam table. "And can you tell him thanks? And that he's the most kick-ass doctor in the world. And that you're the most righteous nurse in the world. And, well, just that I said thankyouthankyouthankyou. . . ."

"I'll tell him." She laughed. "Don't rock too hard tonight."

"No promises."

*　　*　　*

We drove down High Street, looking for the Newport. The street ran straight through the OSU campus, but after a few miles the college kids started looking scummier, so I knew we were close.

On Twelfth, I saw the venue—and a line stretching around the block.

"We're here!" I yelled.

"Fuck yeah!"

"Hurry up and fucking park—fuck!"

We took our place in the back of the unmoving line. I looked at the marquee:

TONITE! PENNYWISE
BOYSETSFIRE DEVIAT3S
SO1D OUT!

I was *here*—in the city, with my favorite band, with my favorite people—it was all so unreal.

"I'm over this waiting around," Nat said. "If you're a VIP, you need to *act* like a VIP—fuck this line, go tell the door guy we're on the list."

"Which list, though?"

"I don't know, man—*the* list. Come on, don't be a chickenshit. Go tell him what's what."

"All right," I said nervously.

I tried not to make eye contact with any other fans as I squeezed past them to the entrance. The door guy looked as if he might squash me.

"Back of the line," he said.

"I think I'm on *the* list."

"Name?"

"It should be."

"I didn't ask what should or shouldn't be," he said. "I asked for your name."

"RUFUS," Nat said loudly behind me. "Rob Rufus, plus one."

The door guy went inside. We stood there shivering for fifteen minutes. I imagined there was some mistake—*of course* we weren't on any list. And now the show was sold out, and I didn't have a ticket. There was no way I'd even get in.

But when he returned, he put his hand on my shoulder.

"Yes sir, you're on there, all right—step this way, please."

The line-waiters cursed as he ushered us inside. He gave us plastic wristbands and told us to go up to the front row of the balcony and wait.

"If you need *anything*," he said, "just flash that wristband and ask."

*   *   *

We sat on the balcony for over an hour. I leaned over the rail as the crowd herded inside. I couldn't see my friends anywhere.

When the opening band came onstage, the club was still filling up with people. By the time Pennywise played, this place was gonna be packed.

"Rob Rufus?" a voice behind us said.

"Yeah," I said, way too eagerly.

He introduced himself as Pennywise's tour manager. He asked us to follow him downstairs. We walked through the crowd, right up to the stage. He banged on a black

355

door with no knob. A security guard opened it, looked at our wristbands, and waved us in.

We walked through the corridors that made up the backstage. We passed the dressing rooms and then went into some type of storage area. From there, we walked out into the alleyway, behind the club.

A tour bus sat there, blowing exhaust through the telephone wires above. The tour manager walked us over.

"Go on up, they're expecting you."

He headed back inside. Nat and I stood there, staring at the door of the bus.

"Come on, VIP," he said.

I laughed nervously and knocked.

The inside of the tour bus wasn't what I'd imagined. It was carpeted in cheesy purple fabric. The counter was covered in potato chips and empty twelve-packs. A TV was on somewhere. I felt more like I was standing in a cramped bachelor pad—only this pad was filled with the members of *one of my favorite bands of all time.*

The band introduced themselves. The roadies didn't bother.

Jim, the singer, wore the same hat he was wearing in the poster on my wall. Randy, the bassist, complimented my Black Flag jacket. Then, we met Fletcher—he stood almost seven feet tall. He wore his hair in a long ponytail, more like a pro wrestler than a musician. He was one of the most infamous punk guitarists alive.

I was intimidated as shit, but they went out of their way to make us feel comfortable. They asked us lots of questions, like you might on a first date. We mostly made small talk about where we were from, our tattoos, our favorite bands.

But a few minutes later, their tour manager came on the bus.

"Thirty minutes till showtime, guys. Time to get rolling!"

The band and crew started grabbing fresh beers and making their way off the bus. Fletcher stood up last. His head almost touched the ceiling.

"Come on, motherfuckers," he said to us. "Let's go give them a show."

I could hear the crowd all the way from backstage.

Not voices—but movement, a rumbling like the place was on the verge of a blowout. The air in the club was thicker now. The molecular structure of the whole damn building was changing.

Fletcher and Randy had their guitars on and stretched their fingers down the frets. Jim paced back and forth. Their drummer was in the dressing room "warming up." Nat and I were trying to stay out of everyone's way.

The tour manager looked at his watch.

"*Five* minutes!"

The band made their way to side stage. Fletcher walked over to me.

"Once we start, you two come watch from the side of the stage—there, near my guitar cab. Cool?"

"Yeah!"

Fletcher nodded—*cool*.

A few minutes later, the stage lights went black.

The crowd let go, erupting into a collective scream

of cusswords and shrieks. The entire room started chanting—*PEN-NY-WISE!*—the ground shook in time with the stomping mob—*PEN-NY-WISE!*—the band ran onto the stage.

"What's up, you motherfuckers!" Fletcher yelled into his mic.

The crowd got even louder.

Jim walked out, mockingly flashing peace signs like Richard Nixon.

"We're Pennywise, from Hermosa Beach. Let's fucking *do this*!"

Nat and I rushed to the corner of the stage, right near the edge. As soon as the band started playing, the entire club spread into a mosh pit—the most violent one I'd ever seen. Kids kicked and punched wildly, boys and girls jumped on and off the stage. Hundreds—*thousands*—of people, screaming the lyrics and losing their minds, were tearing the place apart. I banged my head with the insane volume of the music.

Pennywise blasted through songs without stopping. The room got even hotter. I felt my shirt stick to my chest. The band, the crowd, and the building itself were drenched in the bodyheat chaos of the night.

The band finally took a pause.

"Let me hear you, Ohioooo!" Fletcher yelled.

The crowd yelled back.

"This next song's going out to some friends of ours—two brothers, who are more punk rock than any motherfucker here! *Give it the fuck up!*"

The crowd cheered blindly. Fletcher motioned for us to come onto the stage.

"Holy shit," Nat said.

He grabbed my arm and pulled me under the stage lights. The crowd sounded ten times as loud. I listened for Ali out there, but it was all too crazy.

"Wanna help us sing one?" Fletcher said, and then he turned back toward the crowd. "This one is called *LIV-ING . . . FOR . . . TODAYYYY!*"

The music was all around me. Nat put his arm over my shoulder. He raised a middle finger into the air. I raised my hand and did the same. We stood at the microphone, soaked in spit and sweat, the moment like a perfectly out-of-tune song.

I raised my middle finger higher and began to scream along.

3

After the show, as the bands and crew were winding down, I remembered the demo I had in my pocket. I walked over to the wall that Fletcher leaned against.

"Hey dude," I mumbled, "if y'all get bored on your bus, *or something*, I thought you, like, might wanna check our demo out."

"This is your band?" he asked, looking at the hand-drawn cover.

"Yeah, I mean, me and my bro. He sings and plays guitar, I play drums. This demo is, like, *totally* old, though. We're doing a full-length record in a few months."

"Right on."

"Anyway, if you don't have time to listen to it, it's cool," I said. "We're going to be touring nonstop once our album is done, so maybe you can catch us at a show instead or something. We're way better live, anyways."

"Yeah? You doing any shows in LA?"

I nodded yes.

He took a Sharpie off the table and began writing on a napkin.

"Well, look—here's my cell number and this one is the number to my pad. Give me a shout when you guys are playing, and I'll try to make it out to one of the shows."

I snatched the napkin from his hand. I stared at it.

"Seriously?" I said.

"Shit yeah. Fuck, actually, you know Epitaph?"

"Epitaph *Records*—like, the record label *you guys* are on?"

"Yeah," he said. "Their office is downtown. I'm pretty tight with everyone there, so I'll try to get them to come out and watch you guys play. It couldn't hurt, and they've been pretty much handing out record deals lately."

I was speechless. Literally. Like, I opened my mouth to thank him, but nothing fucking came out.

He took a swig of his beer. I stood there like a mute.

"Well, dude, I guess I'll see ya if you make it out."

TWENTY-SIX

Miracle Child

1

It was Valentine's Day, again.

I had no idea what to do. Things with Ali and me seemed so different. Things had gotten so fucked up. I wasn't sure where I stood. Wherever it was, I doubted that there was a label for it.

Does she still want me to take her out?

Should I buy her candy? Flip the bill? Try to screw her in the car?

Should I just leave her alone?

She might have a date with some other boy, a new one I don't even know about. . . .

I decided to quit being a pussy—just call her, feel it out. . . .

"Happy Valentine's," I said when she answered.

"Ha. Thanks. You too."

"What are you up to?"

"Not much," she said. "Just got home from school. You?"

"Nothin' really. You wanna go, like, get some food?"

She laughed. *"Duh*, I've been waiting for you to ask all week."

I ran into Mom as I headed out the door.

"Where are you off to?"

"Me and Ali are goin' to get something to eat."

"Ooooohhh, you think Cupid will make an appearance?"

"Jesus, Mom."

She smacked me playfully.

"Before you go, I wanted to ask you about the party again."

THE PARTY—*Fuck*. I groaned at the thought.

Mom thought it was finally time to throw a party to celebrate my cancer remission. She'd been pressing me on it for weeks. The idea was okay, in theory . . . but imagining glad-handing a bunch of old classmates and distant relatives—most of whom I'd never even heard from while I was sick—made my skin crawl.

I didn't wanna relive those memories, anyway. I was moving forward, not back.

But Mom wouldn't drop it.

"Mammaw Rufus and your uncle Tony are coming to visit next month, and I know they would love to be there—so I thought maybe we could have it then? We can even call it a 'Fuck Cancer' party if you want, ha-ha."

What she wouldn't ever say was that the party was for her as much as it was for me. The party was for *all of them*—all of the ones who'd stuck. Didn't they warrant some celebrating?

I guessed they probably did.

"Okay—fine," I finally said.

"Yeah?"

"Yeah. Fine. Congratulations, you've suckered me into it. We can do whatever you wanna do, as long as you drop it. Can I go now?"

"*Okay!* Do you need anything? Flowers? Candy?"

"Nah, I think I'd better go unarmed."

*   *   *

We hit the same shitty Mexican joint our first date was at. We sat in the back again, and I could tell that Ali felt as awkward as I did—too much déjà vu to go around, I guess. I asked her about school, but she seemed instantly bored with the topic. All our conversations died on the table.

"Hey," I said, "remember the first time we came here? I was so nervous that all I could talk about was Bon Jovi."

"Of course I remember. And you couldn't have been *that* nervous. I think you're the first boy who's gotten lucky with Jovi trivia since 1985."

I felt my face turn red.

"Have you listened to them lately?" she asked.

"Not really. Have you?"

She shrugged. "I haven't listened to much music at all, really. I'd always just listen to what you were listening to. Now that you haven't needed me nursing you, I've been missin' out on a lot of good tunes."

"Ha-ha. Whatever, Ali. You know I want you nursing me eternally."

"Pshhh," she scoffed, "don't start with that. Just look at you!" She dabbed at her eyes with a napkin. The women in my life were so fucking dramatic. "You've done so good, you've blown me away—I am *so* proud of you. I don't need to take care of my drummer boy anymore."

"Well, what you should really do is start taking care of yourself."

She shrugged. "That's never been my strong suit."

"I'm serious—don't worry about me. Don't worry about your stupid friends, or your parents, or any of that shit—think about what *you* wanna do."

"You know," she said, "lately I've been thinking, maybe I want to work in medicine. Not as a doctor, but maybe a nurse, or maybe I could work with kids. I just wanna, like, help people."

"A *professional* worrier."

She laughed. "Basically. We both know I'm good at that."

We sat there, just looking at each other.

"I think I need a cigarette," she finally said. She grabbed her purse from the chair beside her. "I know, I know—I *am* quitting. Eventually."

I raised my hands. "No judgment, Nurse Wilhelm."

"Smart-ass," she said. But she smiled. "I'll be right back."

She walked past the other tables. I watched her pass families and couples and waiters. None of them looked her way.

How do they not notice her? How can they not stare?

How is that even possible?

I sat there alone, listening to the radio coming from the bar. I waited for a song that I knew would never play.

2

We had almost done it—our tour was almost totally booked.

Every city, every date—one way or another, we were making it work. If no clubs would book us, we found DIY halls like the Y and the VFW. If no DIY promoters wanted us, we found punk kids with basements and absentee parents (thanks to the Internet, it wasn't that hard).

With the recording sessions for our new album starting in just a few weeks, it felt like the stars were actually lining up. Once we got out to California and played for those record label fat cats, we were going to blow them away.

"Yo, big boy," Dad yelled from the top of the basement stairs.

"Yeah?" I turned the stereo down. "What's up?"

Dad walked halfway down and leaned over the railing.

"Come up here for a minute."

"Why?"

"I got you a little 'congratulations' gift," he said. "I wanted to wait and give it to you at the party Saturday, but your brother said if I do it in front of everyone you'll get embarrassed."

"Shit, Dad, you didn't need to do that. What is it?"

"Get your lazy ass upstairs and see for yourself. Meet me in the backyard. Nat has it stashed in the garage."

"Remember, this isn't as much a gift as it is a project," Dad said. "Now that you aren't lying in bed all day, you need something to do with your time. A man has got to stay busy."

"I mean, that's cool, but . . . I don't know if I have time for a project. We're about to do the new record, and Mom said that school might even let me come back for the last few months of the semester. I don't think I'll have time for a bunch of extra work."

"Trust me," he said, "it's not that kind of work."

We walked through the yard and into the alley. The garage door was open.

Nat stood silhouetted against it.

The car.

It was the car from the lot in Ohio. It was the cherry-red convertible. It was the raised Avenger tires. It was the '68 Mustang. It was the Springsteen song.

It was the car!

"No way. Nofuckingway!" I yelled.

The two of them started clapping.

I walked into the garage, totally stunned. I ran my hand against the paint. It was warm.

"It's still a piece-of-shit car," Dad said, "but you loved it so much and, screw it. I only have two kids."

"This is *so* not a piece-of-shit car," I said again.

Nat laughed. "Actually, it kinda is. It broke down about eight times on the way home. Took like three hours. But I gotta say, this thing is rock 'n' roll as hell."

"I don't know if I can take this."

They both ignored me.

"She needs a new carb, and new rear brakes," Dad said. "She's been leaking fluid, but I can't tell what. Still has the original engine, though—an old two-eighty-nine."

I had no idea what any of that meant.

"We'll have your uncle Tony look at it after the party," he said. "He'll be able to help fix it up, maybe."

"Can I drive it?" I asked.

"If it'll start."

Nat climbed into the backseat. Dad took shotgun. I grabbed the steering wheel nervously. I'd never been inside anything like this before.

I turned the key. The engine *clickclickclickclicked*, but then nothing. I looked over at Dad.

"Pump the gas a few times," he said. "But don't flood the engine. And be careful with the steering, it's different than the van."

I turned the key again.

This time, the motor turned over—the noise was so loud that my ears popped. It *ROARED* to life! Smoke shot out of the exhaust pipes, filling the garage.

The engine growled while the car rumbled in place, shaking like an untamed animal. I could feel those shakes in my bones. I shifted into reverse and hit the gas too hard. The car shot into the alley. I turned the wheel and slammed on the brakes. Dad jerked into the dash.

The engine died.

"Jesus," Nat yelled.

"This is awesome!" I said. I turned the ignition again.

The car came back to life. I floored it down the alleyway. Smoke clouds followed us into the street.

The smell of oil came through the floor. I clicked on the radio, but I could barely hear it above the engine.

The speedometer trembled in place. Dad said it was

broken. I had no clue how fast I was going . . . only that I wanted to go faster.

Faster! Forward! Faster! Forward! The words lit up in dashboard green.

I gripped the wheel harder and pushed the accelerator down.

3

Look, I wish the story wrapped up right there. Me on a cancer-free joyride in the car of my dreams, the sun shining on a horizon holding a record deal, a tour, and a kick-ass party surrounded by all my friends and family. I can almost see the photo from that pretend moment. All of us standing in the front yard, my bitchin' Mustang next to us in the driveway. And we're all smiling, waving at the camera. Yeah, that would have been great. It would have been fucking touching, even.

It's just, that's not what happened.

The car stalled out three more times before Dad made me drive it home. I could feel the engine struggling, chugging and coughing along in the same way that I did. I backed into the garage slowly, trying not to nick the paint.

Mom must have heard us arrive (the whole fucking neighborhood probably heard us arrive) as she was standing outside, waiting for us.

"Mom!" I yelled. "Look at it!"

She smiled weakly. "It's cool, all right. Pretty awesome."

"Mom, it's *amazing*," I said, my excitement blinding me to what was coming. "You *have* to take a ride! Seriously."

A sigh passed her lips. She looked at my dad. "Columbus just called. They need us to drive up tomorrow—can you take off work and come with me?"

My stomach instantly tensed. I was listening now.

"What?" I asked. "My next appointment isn't for three weeks."

"They want you to come in anyway," Mom said.

"But *why*?"

"I don't know, honey."

"Bullshit," I snapped. "What is it? Tell me. It can't be *good* news—if it was something like that Pennywise show, they woulda said."

"But that doesn't mean it's something *bad*," Dad said. "It's illegal for them to discuss medical stuff on the phone, that's all. That's the only reason they asked us to come up. It's probably nothing."

Nat was standing in the garage, looking at the three of us and not sure what to say.

I moaned and let the air out of my sail. I leaned on the hood of my getaway car. Although I knew the engine was dead, I swear I felt shaking beneath my hands.

4

Talk from the radio filled the silence between us. Dad and Mom sat up front, faking interest about a news story, trying to seem relaxed.

Something was up. I had no clue what I was walking into, and it made me nervous as hell.

Did they have a new machine to scan me with? Was there another horrible test to run? What if I needed another surgery? I hadn't worried about my health in so long—now I felt like I'd been kidding myself.

Why the hell did they call me back to this place?

* * *

We were the only ones in the oncology clinic. It was early, and most of the nurses were just now showing up for their shifts. I sat there waiting for my name to be called, dumbly praying that it wouldn't be.

"Robert Rufus?"

My parents stood up and walked toward the nurse. I stayed plastered in my chair. I didn't want to hear whatever they had to say to me. I wanted to be left alone.

Mom motioned me over. I sat stubbornly. She pointed sternly at the ground—finally, like a meek dog, I obeyed.

We waited.

You wait in a room just to wait in a room, I remembered saying.

It didn't seem so clever anymore. I sat on the edge of the exam table, kicking my feet nervously.

There was a tap on the door.

Dr. Ranalli and Stacey walked in. Stacey wore a tight red turtleneck sweater. She looked good. But Dr. Ranalli looked just plain exhausted. He rolled the stool from the counter and sat down with a groan.

"Okay," he said, trying to sound upbeat, "so—we noticed something strange on Robert's last PET scan. What looks like a recurrence seems to have developed in your right calf *and* in your left hip."

I looked at my leg. I looked at my side.

"What does that *mean*?" Mom asked. "A recurrence? Are you saying he has to get more chemotherapy?"

"I can't say exactly what it means," he said. "We need to schedule some biopsies. But the markers in his blood count have increased too—first negligibly, but now, well, the fact that the PET scan registered this, after an entire *year* of treatments and surgery, is extremely concerning to me. *Not* hopeless—but concerning. The fact that it's recurred in new areas of the body suggests that the disease is even more thoroughly progressed."

"More progressed than Stage Four cancer?" Mom asked.

Dr. Ranalli cleared his throat.

"There is a new chemo cocktail that's showed promising signs in Japan recently, although we've never used that combination of drugs here before. The treatment entails lower doses, over a much longer period of time, as well as radiation therapy."

We all just sat there.

"But you've never tried it before," Dad said. "So what if this new treatment doesn't work? What's our plan B here? Surgery?"

"No," Dr. Ranalli said, "not surgery. We should be able to gauge the effectiveness of the therapy around the third session."

"If it isn't effective," Stacey interrupted, looking at me, "we have other medications that will keep you comfortable."

Her words took up the entire room.

"*Comfortable*—what does that even *mean*?" I said. "Like,

that's it? Like, some fucking Japanese drugs don't work, and now I'm going to fucking *die*? I don't *want* to be comfortable! *No one wants to be fucking comfortable!*"

I felt my heart racing wildly. I grabbed my knee.

"The cancer came back in my leg? *Cut my fucking leg off!* I don't care! *But don't fucking tell me you can make me* comfortable. *Don't tell* me that, man. Please."

Mom clasped her hand over her mouth.

Dr. Ranalli leaned closer to me. He laid his hand on my knee, as if to steady me.

"Rob, look, I know this is bad news," he said, "believe me, I know. But you've *got* to remember that your situation *isn't* hopeless. You still have a chance. For a guy like you, a chance is all you need."

I didn't say anything. I was out of words.

I was empty.

5

"But they're already on their way," Mom said. "I literally have no way to tell them not to come, honey."

I was hunched in the backseat.

"So I'm supposed to sit at a 'party' where a bunch of assholes come and feel sorry for me? I feel like I'm going to my own funeral."

"That isn't funny," Dad said.

Mom turned around to face me. "I know that 'bad timing' doesn't even come close to nailing this, but these people are only coming because they care about you."

"Fuck them," I snapped.

Dad turned onto our block. My Mustang sat on the

curb, glistening under our oak trees. Nat must have moved it so the partygoers could cast jealous glances at it.

"Goddammit," I said. "*At least* don't say anything about this news—okay? Even to Nat. Just tell him I'm waiting on a test result or something. I don't care. But no one can know. I won't be able to fucking handle it if they know."

With that, I opened the door and hurled myself toward the house like a cannonball ready to explode.

6

Everyone seemed to be having a good time at my fake just-beat-cancer party. The house was filled with guests—mostly relatives, standing in the backyard drinking Coronas and talking about boring adult stuff. Dad's Sam Cooke LP was spinning.

My parents were doing a fine job of playing hosts. I was the only one who noticed the way they avoided people's eyes. Old women came up to hug me. Strangers shook my hand and slapped my shoulder. I stood there lifelessly, taking it. I was exhausted in the very core of my being.

I stayed in the kitchen with my friends.

I watched as Doyle and Tyson scarfed down countless slices of pizza. Paul was pulling a Cool Hand Luke, trying to see how many slices he could shove into his mouth at once—he was up to three. Ali sat at the table, laughing hysterically at him. Her nose crinkled, making the freckles on her cheeks light up. She must have been stoned.

How am I supposed to tell them that I have cancer again?

Life was finally back on track—now I was supposed

to drag them back into my bullshit? And the band? The tour. The album. The record deal. *Everything* was ruined.

They just didn't know it yet.

I looked back at Ali. She looked so perfect when she laughed. She brushed her hand through her hair carelessly.

I sighed and shut my eyes.

"Hey there, sweetheart," a voice said cheerfully.

I looked at a small woman with curly white hair. She held her hands out eagerly.

"I'm your great-aunt Liza," she said, "Margie's sister. You 'member me? I haven't seen y'all since you were just little bitty things."

She put her arms around me in a weak hug. She looked up at me, rubbing my shoulders.

"Margie told me 'bout the party, and I just wanted to come and tell y'all how thankful we all are that you had such a blessed recovery."

"Thanks."

"Did Margie tell you our congregation prayed for you? Every Sunday, twice a day, we did. Yep."

"Great," I mumbled. "Tell everyone thanks."

"How happy they'd be to see you standing here like this. You're our little miracle child."

"No," I mumbled. "I'm not."

She smiled warmly. "But you are. God has *saved* you—his grace has shined on *you*."

"Just please shut the fuck up," I snapped without thinking.

Paul coughed on his pizza. She stepped backward, shocked.

I pushed past all of them. I stumbled away. All the oxygen had drained from the house. I felt like my heart was about to explode.

I pushed through the front door.

I steadied myself on the front porch railing, fighting for breath. It was all too much. I couldn't think. I couldn't deal. Not with this—not again.

"You all right?" Nat said. I hadn't realized he was out there. I wasn't sure I could handle him being there at that moment.

I shook my head. I was about to tell him, but I would have just started crying right there.

I finally pulled my shit together and managed a weak "I'm fine, man."

"Well—you want to go cruise?"

"Right now?"

He shrugged again. "Why not? It's your party—you can bail if you want to."

I pulled the keys from the pocket of my jeans. Nat snatched them from my hand.

"No way," he said. "I'm driving this time. You look like you're about to keel the fuck over. Come on."

He put his hand around my shoulder, steadying me as we walked through the yard. My breath was slowly coming back. Nat opened the passenger door and I slid in. The leather was warm underneath me. The dying sun cast a bright orange glare through the windshield. I strained my eyes into the firelight.

Nat put down the convertible top. And this time, the engine turned over on the first shot.

The roar of the 289 killed any thoughts in my head.

Nat put the pedal to the floor. We blasted through our neighborhood, past the park, past the school, and onto the empty highway.

The mountains swallowed the horizon before us and the sky dimmed overhead. I leaned back and let the air wash over the remains of my broken body. Tears stung at my eyes. Nat didn't notice. The wind carried them into the night.

"So where do you wanna go?" my brother asked.

"I don't know," I said. "Anywhere. Everywhere. I just don't want to stop. I'm not ready to. *I'm just not ready to stop.*"

The road stretched out through the small towns before us, toward the cities and skylines I knew lay ahead. The road stretched across those deserts beyond them, over all the empty space. The road stretched out into the nothing, to the place where the sky was blacker than black.

We moved faster now, away from it all. The road stretched farther away from my pain and straight into my undying basement dreams, where bright red stars lit a path up to heaven, and all the midnight girls of Hamburg sparkled under pink lights out in the streets.

EPILOGUE

And we never did stop.

Through the cancer coming back, through the pain, through chemo, radiation, and every ounce of bad luck under the sun, we never stopped.

I don't think we even knew how.

I was finally considered cancer-free two months before my twenty-fifth birthday, five years after the last of the chemo was administered into my bloodstream. I spent that day with my brother, somewhere out on the West Coast. We celebrated by playing rock 'n' roll.

Blacklist Royals—the band we formed from the ashes of Defiance of Authority—was touring constantly by then, covering ground like it was going out of style. The hospital's shadow still loomed heavily across those years, and the only shelter we found was the road. So we played hundreds of shows in dive bars and basements all over North America.

Each performance was a form of recompense, but it was never enough.

As of today, we've toured in over eleven countries, and shared the stage with all of the bands that we worshipped when we were kids. I've played punk rock music with my twin brother all over the goddamn world.

In 2014, we put out *Die Young with Me*, an album that grappled with each of our battles over those years, shit we hadn't even talked to each other about. We couldn't. But turned out we could make music about it—go figure, right?

The record got love from critics, but a lot of our fans thought it was too sad. You can't please everyone, I guess, but at least we got enough buzz to play on TV. Not too bad for a dumb crippled punk, if I do say so myself.

I live in Nashville now, in a little ranch house over on the East Side. It's nice here, big-city enough for good tours to come through, but still redneck enough to feel like home. My hallway is covered in photos and flyers, keepsakes from our tours and travels. *Goddamn,* I think to myself sometimes, *we really did it, didn't we?*

But the walls of my bedroom tell a different story. The photos in there are faded and old, some torn and crammed into frames. Nat, Paul, and me in my hospital room. Onstage, singing with Pennywise. Mom and Dad on my eighteenth birthday.

And Ali. Of course, there's always Ali.

Black-and-white smiles shine down from that old photo, still in its frame, tacked up on my wall. Me and Ali. Ali and me. Us, on that bad day, the day that it all changed.

Us, in another life.

We still talk on the phone, some nights. She comes to

see me when I play down in Pensacola or New Orleans, or whatever port town she happens to live in at the time. She moves around a lot with her fiancé, an offshore oil-rig worker whom I still can't believe she digs.

Ah well. At least she got out. Tyson got out of there too—like I told you, he was always the smart one.

Some of the others, though, they weren't so lucky.

Doyle did okay for himself back home, all in all; he stocks shelves at the Sam's Club down off Route 60. I heard Brody got a job selling insurance. He still keeps talking about starting up his own band.

But hopelessness is a birthright in West Virginia, as easy to slip into as a warm bath. It doesn't matter who you are—if you stay there long enough, you see what's on the dark side of those mountains.

I lost so many old friends because of it. Those sweet, bright kids who never hurt a damn fly. Most of them overdosed. Some of them meant to. The rest of 'em just drifted down into the nothing.

And Paul—*goddammit, Paul.*

Paul got hooked on Oxy, just like the rest. It wasn't his fault—he broke his hand in a fistfight (his punches were always too damn wild) and got a prescription from the doctor who fixed him up. That hooked him in. That was all it took.

A few months later he ended up in jail, but Nat and I got word and bailed him out. Last time I saw him was Christmas Day, four years ago. He stole all the pills in my medicine bag. I haven't heard from him since. I heard he's cleaned up now, but I really couldn't say.

But man, I miss him sometimes.

I miss all of them, my skeleton crew. I still see them so clearly in my mind, jumping and dancing to the punk-rock racket that blasts from our basement stereo. I see us bombing Fifth Avenue hill on our skateboards. I see Ali, smiling her smile for me, for nobody else but me.

People say it's unhealthy to live in the past. But what choice do I have when it defines my every moment? It's with me when I hurt, when I struggle for breath. It's written on my skin, in scars and tattoos. It's in the '68 Mustang that's broken down in my driveway. It's in everything I do. It's all around me, always.

But fuck it, that's all right.

I don't mind the past too much.

After all, it had one hell of a soundtrack.

ACKNOWLEDGMENTS

My wonderful agent and dreamweaver, Shannon Hassan, for her unwavering belief in a cynical, foulmouthed first-time author like me. Shannon's wit, perseverance, and empathetic spirit took this project to places I never imagined it could go.

My badass editor, Matthew Benjamin, for taking a chance on me. Matthew helped turn my insane, rambling manuscript into a coherent, digestible thought—all while keeping its spirit intact. He's been my steady captain through these unfamiliar waters of the literary world, and he hasn't steered me wrong yet.

Brooke Warner, who coached and encouraged me during my first days of writing. Funny how a little validation can keep you from putting down the pen.

Everyone at Touchstone Books and Simon & Schuster, for working so ridiculously hard on this project. Drinks are on me, y'all.

My family, for their unwavering belief in the strength

of will, the power of knowledge, and the value of art. I love you guys big-time.

All those who appeared in *Die Young with Me,* and all those who didn't but should've. Your presence in my life has been invaluable. Thank you for joining me on my disjointed, nostalgia-fueled morphine dream of the past.

ABOUT THE AUTHOR

Rob Rufus is a musician, songwriter, author, and activist living in Nashville, Tennessee. He is the cofounder of Blacklist Royals, a punk rock band that's garnered worldwide acclaim throughout the past decade. His new project, The Bad Signs, released their first single on Halloween of 2015. Rob remains passionate within the cancer community and has collaborated with Make-A-Wish Foundation, Livestrong Foundation, Stupid Cancer, Imerman Angels, Gilda's Club, and more. His articles have appeared in *Modern Drummer, Amp Magazine, Digital Tour Bus*, and various music and culture websites. He is currently at work on his second book.